HELP! WHAT VITAMINS SHOULD I TAKE FOR MY EYES?

The Easy Guide to Eye Nutrition

Keith Ngan MRPharmS

Help! What Vitamins Should I Take for My Eyes?
The Easy Guide to Eye Nutrition

www.IntelligentFormula.co.uk

Readers should be aware that websites and publications listed in this work may have changed between when this work was written, and when it is read.

Disclaimer: While this book examines the research supporting nutrients and herbal remedies for ocular health, it is for information only. Reasonable efforts have been made to publish reliable data and information, but the author and publisher cannot assume responsibility for the validity of all materials or the consequences of their use. This book is not intended to diagnose, treat, cure, or prevent any disease. Before taking any supplements or changing your diet, first consult your doctor or a suitably qualified healthcare professional. While this book was developed with ocular health in mind, consuming supplements or changing your diet should not replace regular eye health examinations by a qualified optometrist or ophthalmologist.

For my beloved wife and family.

*Above all, to Him who can truly
open blind eyes...*

CONTENTS

INTRODUCTION

Vision is probably the most treasured of the five senses. When your eyesight becomes blurred or is completely lost, it is hard to concentrate on anything beyond the health of your eyes. This book will empower you to understand the inner workings of the eye as well as the nutrients needed for maintaining optimal function and longevity. From age-related macular degeneration through to conjunctivitis, glaucoma to dry eyes, we will address the most common eye conditions and explore effective evidence-based nutritional and herbal therapies.

The information in this book is based on high-quality peer-reviewed research in conjunction with traditional or historical usage. Where possible, we have included references and links to the relevant research so you can find out more. We have designed this book so that you can 'dip in and out' as necessary. This means that some information may be repeated – apologies if you're reading from cover to cover!

We caution you that getting a clear diagnosis is the first step in finding effective treatment – there's no point using therapies for conjunctivitis when you have a case of blepharitis! Always seek diagnostic support from a medical professional before taking natural remedies and supplements. We have highlighted the most essential cautions and possible side effects, but always seek personalised advice from a qualified nutritionist, naturopath, or integrative doctor. Do NOT hesitate to see a medical professional if you experience allergic reactions or worsening symptoms after taking a supplement or natural therapy.

Knowledge is power, so let's begin with an overview of the main structures of the eye, how they fit together and their physiological roles. After this, we'll dive into a detailed explanation of the underlying processes that can cause dysfunction and disease in the eyes.

1. QUICK GUIDE TO EYE ANATOMY & PHYSIOLOGY

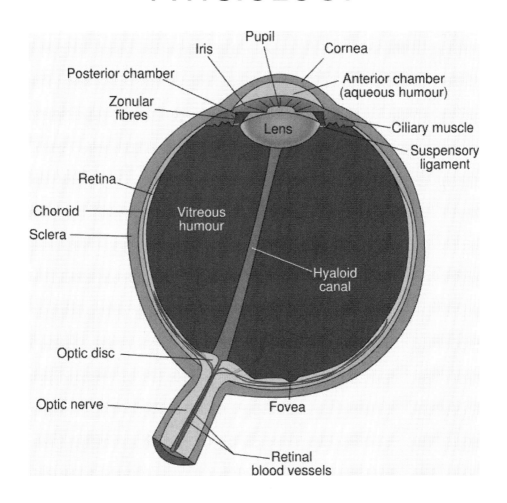

1. General Features of the Eye

The outer layer of the eye is the **cornea**.

The interior of the eye is divided into two segments: the anterior ('front') and posterior ('back') segments.

The front segment contains the **cornea, iris, ciliary body**, and **lens** as well as aqueous humour – a transparent watery substance that is released from the skin-like covering of the **ciliary body**.

The back segment of the eye contains the **retina, macula, optic nerve head**, and a compartment filled with a jelly-like substance called the **vitreous humour**.

A thin membrane called the **conjunctiva** wraps around the front of the eyeball, over the cornea, and lines the internal surface of the eyelids.

2. Basic Eye Physiology

Light enters the eye and is, mostly, focussed by the **cornea.** This is the clear surface at the front of the eye. You could consider this to be a 'camera lens', as it captures the light that is aimed at it.

By adjusting the size of the pupil, the **iris** controls the amount of light that reaches the back of the eye. Right behind the pupil is the **lens.** This is a crystal-like structure that further focusses light and directs it towards the back of the eye. In a process called 'accommodation', the muscles of the **ciliary body** flex to control the shape of the lens so it can take in different amounts of light to automatically focus on nearby, or approaching, objects.

This focussed light moves towards the back of the eye. It reaches the **retina,** a nerve layer that acts like an electronic sensor. The retina converts light or optical images (what you 'see') into electrical signals. These electrical signals are then sent via the **optic nerve** to the part of the brain that controls the sense of sight – the **visual cortex**.

The **macula** is a small area of light-sensitive cells in the retina. Macular cells are tuned to detect fine-detailed light. The macula is a very important part of the eye. It is responsible for our central vision (as opposed to peripheral, or side, vision) and most of our colour vision and vision of fine details.

Within the macula is a layer of **macular pigment** which acts as a protective shield. It catches certain dangerous wavelengths of blue light and stops them from damaging the retina. Healthy macular pigment improves the eye's ability to pick up on the contrast between dark and light and stops a blue haze from appearing around objects. The **macular pigment** is a layer of coloured pigment that is made up of **carotenoids – lutein, zeaxanthin**, and **meso-zeaxanthin.** These carotenoids are yellow, so they are able to absorb blue light that would otherwise damage the macular nerves and alter vision. The carotenoids also have antioxidant properties which help to protect the eye.

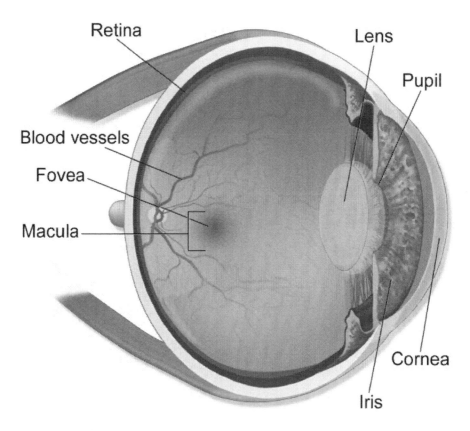

Image showing location of the macula (Source: Blausen.com staff)

3. Quick Reference Guide

Ciliary Body: Contains muscles that control the size and shape of the **lens** to automatically focus light coming from the **cornea**.

Cornea: The 'camera lens' of the eye. Positioned at the front of the eye where it captures light and directs it towards the **lens.**

Iris: The coloured part of the eye that helps to focus light by adjusting the size of the **pupil**.

Lens: The transparent structure located behind the **pupil** that further focusses light onto the retina.

Macula: A small area in the **retina** that contains light-sensitive cells for fine-detailed vision and central vision.

Macular Pigment: A layer of macular carotenoids (**lutein, zeaxanthin**, and **meso-zeaxanthin**) that filters blue light waves and protects the **macula** and **retina**.

Optic Nerve: The nerve that carries electrical impulses from the **retina** to the brain to be interpreted as images.

Pupil: The dark centre at the front of the eye, surrounded by the **iris** and located behind the **cornea**.

Retina: A layer of nerve tissue at the back of the eye that detects light and converts it into electrical impulses to be sent through the **optic nerve** to the brain.

2. COMMON THEMES IN EYE HEALTH & DISEASE

1. Oxidative Stress
2. Electrolyte Imbalances
3. Glycation & Lens Protein Changes
4. Hyperglycaemia
5. Microcirculation Issues

1. Oxidative Stress

Oxidative stress is a major cause of damage to the eyes, but what is it exactly? You may have heard about free radicals – molecules that *freely* attack other molecules and cause *radical* negative changes to the stability and function of cells. Understanding these chemical interactions can help us to understand the basis of oxidative stress and how it affects the health of eye tissues.

Time for a quick chemistry refresher. Don't worry, we'll keep it simple!

An atom has protons and neutrons at its centre and these are orbited by electrons. [Science has discovered that there is a deeper level of quarks and quantum physics involved in this process, but their effects on eye health are not yet fully understood, so will not discuss this here!].

The interaction of electrons between different atoms creates chemical reactions. When electrons bond atoms together, they form molecules. Many molecules combine to form cells, and these cells form the tissues of the human body, including the eyes.

Zooming back to the molecular level, we can imagine atoms as having shells that electrons orbit around. Each shell is only able to hold a set number of electrons. If the outer shell of an atom contains its maximum number of electrons, then that atom is considered **stable** – think of it as being happy, fulfilled, and unlikely to interact with other atoms.

However, an atom is considered **unstable** when the outermost shell contains some electrons, but it isn't full. The electrons in the unfilled outer shell are **unpaired**. All atoms want to be stable and they'll do anything to get that way (Lobo, et al., 2010; Pham-Huy, et al., 2008).

An unstable atom with unpaired electrons will do one of three things, depending on the number of electrons and which shell is involved:
1. It may give away electrons so that its outer shell becomes empty. This makes the next-shell-down a full shell, and the atom becomes stable again
2. It may take electrons from other atoms to fill its outer shell, becoming stable again
3. It may bond with another atom by sharing electrons with it, forming a **molecule**

Here's where free radicals come in!

Atoms that are bonded together as molecules don't *usually* split apart in a way that leaves an unpaired electron floating around in an outer shell. But it does happen – weak bonds split and result in unstable, highly reactive molecules called **free radicals.** These molecules are volatile and have a very strong charge. Free radicals will react with the nearest molecule and steal its electron. The molecule it reacts with will lose an electron from its outer shell in this exchange and become a free radical itself. This process cascades from molecule to molecule and can eventually disrupt the function of a living cell; free radical cascades affect lipids, proteins, and DNA within the body, including in the eyes.

The human body always has a degree of free radical activity. These reckless molecules are usually kept in check by **antioxidant nutrients** and enzymes. Usually...

Oxidative stress refers to an imbalance of free radical activity in the body. When free radical cascades overpower the available reserves of antioxidants, cellular damage is unstoppable, cellular health is impaired, and cellular death can even result. As the cascade continues, a large number of cells are affected and the health of the body's tissues or organs can become compromised. An escalation of oxidative stress naturally occurs as the body ages, but further acceleration can cause disease.

Common sources of free radicals and oxidative stress in the eyes include:
- Ultraviolet (UV) light damage, particularly from blue light waves
- Infection by any bacteria, virus, or parasite
- Accumulation of **advanced glycation end products** (Gillery, 2001)
- **Electrolyte imbalances**
- Toxic effects of cigarette smoke, including passive smoke exposure
- The natural ageing processes
- Inadequate antioxidant intake through the diet (Sievert, 2017)

Oxidative stress has been associated with **lens protein changes** leading to the formation of **cataracts,** optic nerve damage found in **glaucoma**, impaired rod sensitivity in **nyctalopia** (night blindness), the accumulation of fatty deposits in **age-related macular degeneration,** changes to tear composition that can cause **dry eye syndrome,** and inflammation in **conjunctivitis** and **blepharitis**

(Kruk, et al., 2015).

2. Electrolyte Imbalances

Electrolytes are salts that carry an electrical charge. Some of the most important electrolytes are **sodium**, **potassium**, **magnesium**, and **calcium**. The cells in the eyes rely on these electrolytes to control communication between cells and to pass on the electrical changes needed for nerve signals and muscle contractions. Without a proper balance of electrolytes, cellular communication pathways can break down.

Sodium-potassium pumps (Na+/K- pumps) exist in the membranes (or 'walls') of most cells in the eye tissues. The purpose of a sodium-potassium pump is to carry an electrical charge across the membrane by trading positively charged sodium ions for negatively charged potassium ions. Positive for negative. This exchange creates energy that can be used as an electrical signal. Disturbances to sodium levels (either too much or too little sodium) will interfere with this exchange and with the eye cells' ability to receive and send nerve signals. If the disturbance lasts a long time or is severe, it can paralyse the cells' transport and communication systems, and eventually lead to cell death.

Disturbances to the sodium-potassium pump and cellular electrical signals have been associated with optic nerve damage in **glaucoma** and lens protein changes associated with **cataracts.**

A functioning sodium-potassium pump and a healthy ratio of the two minerals is essential for a balance of sodium inside and outside the cell. Sodium also influences the hydration of the cell. Where sodium goes, water flows – if there is more sodium within a cell than outside it, fluid will flow into the cell and cause it to become swollen and, eventually, burst! Too little sodium inside the cell, or too much in the fluid surrounding it, will draw liquid from inside the cell. This can dehydrate the cell and crush the structures found inside.

> Too much sodium outside the cell = the cell becomes dried up and crushed.

Too much sodium inside the cell = the cell fills up with water and bursts.

The proper balance of electrolytes also affects fluids outside of the cells. **Tear osmolarity** refers to the number of electrolytes found within the tear fluids. In normal human tear fluid, **sodium**, **potassium**, **calcium**, and **magnesium** are in perfect balance. In conditions such as **dry eye syndrome**, the concentration of these electrolytes increases. Tear film is designed to help protect the surface of the eye. High tear osmolarity (or 'hyper-osmolarity') means that there is a high concentration of electrolytes and a low level of liquid. With a scarce amount of liquid, the tear film quickly evaporates or dries out. As well as leading to symptoms of **dry eye syndrome**, this electrolyte imbalance and fast evaporation contributes to damage to the ocular (eye) surface. The high concentration of electrolytes in the evaporating tear film pulls water out of the cells, leading to cellular dehydration and eventual cell death (Januleviciene, et al., 2012; Woodward, et al., 2014).

Proper electrolyte balance is essential for the flow of water-soluble molecules into and out of the cells of the eyes. For example, when there is an electrolyte imbalance, antioxidants are unable to flow into areas like the nuclei of cells in the lens. When antioxidants are unable to reach these important areas of the eye's cells, free radicals can cause unstoppable damage and lead to severe **oxidative stress**. In short, electrolyte imbalances can stop antioxidants from addressing oxidative stress, which causes damage to proteins (e.g. **lens protein changes**) and leads to conditions such as **cataracts** (Cumming, et al., 2000).

Electrolyte imbalances are also implicated in **age-related macular degeneration** (Bringmann, et al., 2016).

Electrolyte imbalances can be caused by:
- Certain medications, including diuretics and chemotherapy (check with your pharmacist or doctor)
- Kidney damage or disease
- Illnesses involving vomiting, diarrhoea, fever, and

sweating
- Poor diet with high sodium intake and low levels of other electrolytes
- Digestive conditions that stop the absorption of some or all electrolytes

3. Glycation & Lens Protein Changes

The lens is responsible for the fine-focussing of light onto the retina, and it is essential that the lens remains transparent if vision is to remain accurate.

Around 33% of the weight of the lens is made of proteins. These proteins make up the lens **crystallins** as well as other structures, such as cellular skeletons (think of these as being similar to the foundations of a house), membrane proteins (the 'walls' of the house), and transporters that carry things into, out of, and within the cell. Crystallins are very stable, tightly folded proteins that have a number of roles in the cornea and lens – in particular, they maintain lens transparency. They control the direction that light flows into and through the eye. This is called the 'refractive index'.

Glycation

Changes to crystallins and other key lens proteins are believed to begin with glycation, which occurs when proteins are exposed to simple **carbohydrates** – sugars. Glycation is a process where a sugar aldehyde group interacts with groups of amino acids in the proteins. To keep it simple, sugar initiates the unfolding of the tightly bound protein structure. Once the protein's structure is unfolded, it is susceptible to free radical attack and **oxidative stress.** These attacks break off pieces of the crystallin molecules and other key proteins, creating 'denatured proteins' and oxidised crystallin fragments. Over time, these fragments can clump together in the lens, causing the lens to take on a white-grey opacity. This contributes to the formation of **cataracts.**

When the glycation of proteins and lipids occurs in other parts of the eye, it can lead to the destruction of the trabecular meshwork (responsible for draining aqueous humour from the eye), as seen in **glaucoma**; damage to the lacrimal (tear) gland, as seen in **dry eye syndrome**; and changes to the opacity of the lens, as seen in **cataracts** (Alves, et al., 2005; Howes, et al., 2004; Michael & Bron, 2011).

4. Hyperglycaemia

As discussed above, **glycation** is initiated by sugar. The sugars that cause high levels of glycation are delivered into the eye tissues via the circulatory system. Hyperglycaemia is a state of too much glucose (sugar) in the blood – when there is too much sugar in the blood, there will be a correspondingly high level of sugar in the eye tissues.

Causes of hyperglycaemia include:
- Type 1 diabetes, where there is an insufficient amount of insulin to pull the glucose into cells and out of the blood. Type 1 diabetes is an autoimmune condition that cannot be reversed but can be managed with medication, lifestyle, and diet
- Type 2 diabetes, where there are adequate amounts of insulin, but cells are resistant to its actions and leave lots of glucose in the blood. Many cases of type 2 diabetes have been reversed with changes to nutrition, lifestyle, and diet (Lim, et al., 2011)
- Medications such as corticosteroids, beta-blockers, and statins
- High-dose **niacin** (vitamin B3)
- Critical illness, such as stroke or heart attack
- Certain types of tumours
- Stress, especially ongoing stress or acute emotional trauma
- Issues with the thyroid gland, adrenal gland, or pituitary gland
- Pancreatic diseases
- Diseases that affect the brain, such as meningitis, en-

cephalitis, and brain tumours

With high levels of glucose in the blood, **glycation** and the oxidation of proteins and lipids in the eye becomes more likely. Hyperglycaemia can also initiate the swelling of lens fibres, increase **oxidative stress,** reduce tear film quality, and lower the eye's immune defences. It can result in damage to the nerves and blood vessels of the eyes and has been associated with an increased risk of **glaucoma, cataracts, dry eye syndrome, blepharitis**, and **age-related macular degeneration** (Calvo-Maroto, et al., 2014; Chen, et al., 2014; Boptom & Braavedt, 2015).

5. Microcirculation Issues

The tissues and cells of the eyes are supplied with oxygen and nutrients via a network of tiny blood vessels. The major arteries that supply the eye with blood are only about 2mm in diameter! These arteries branch off into even smaller capillaries which supply blood, oxygen, and nutrients to the muscles that move the eye, the eyelid, and the cells of the eyeball itself. This is called 'microcirculation'.

The ophthalmic veins and central retinal veins drain blood from the eye and carry away debris, toxins, and waste products.

The steady, regular, and healthy flow of blood to and from the eye is essential for its health and function. Blood flowing in from the arteries brings oxygen and nutrients required for the production of cellular energy, but also brings hormones, proteins, and other chemical messengers that help to regulate eye health. Blood is also full of immune cells that protect the eye tissues against infection. Any disruption to the steady, abundant flow of blood to the eyes can lead to a lack of oxygen, huge amounts of **oxidative stress**, cell death, and tissue dysfunction. Chronic diseases of the eyes tend to develop over many years, so issues with microcirculation can go completely unnoticed.

Major causes of microcirculation dysfunction include:

- **Oxidative stress** – can directly damage the blood vessels

- **Hyperglycaemia** – large sugar molecules in the blood can damage the internal lining of blood vessels. How this occurs is still unknown, but researchers suspect that **glycation** and **oxidative stress** are responsible (Peppa, et al., 2003)
- High cholesterol – cholesterol can become lodged in micro blood vessels or in larger arteries, leading to an 'occlusion' or partial blockage that stops smooth blood flow into the microcirculation of the eyes
- High blood pressure – the pressure within the blood vessels can damage the vessels themselves, leading to partial occlusion or blockage
- Contraction and relaxation issues – the blood flow in microcirculation depends on a process called vasomotion (the rhythmic contraction and relaxation of the small muscles at either end of the tiny eye capillaries). Think of these muscles as pumps. Issues with vasomotion can occur due to nerve damage, improper nerve signalling, and **electrolyte imbalances**

3. NUTRIENTS FOR EYE HEALTH

1. Vitamin A & Carotenoids
2. B-Group Vitamins
3. Vitamin C
4. Vitamin D
5. Vitamin E
6. Magnesium
7. Sodium
8. Zinc
9. Omega-3 Essential Fatty Acids
10. Omega-7 Fatty Acids
11. Carbohydrates
12. Quercetin

1. Vitamin A & Carotenoids

Vitamin A and all carotenoids are fat-soluble. This means that they must be consumed at the same time as dietary fat or they won't be absorbed through the small intestines and into the body.

Vitamin A

Vitamin A is used by every cell in the body for growth and many basic cellular functions. It is an essential nutrient for eye health. A deficiency in vitamin A can cause **keratomalacia.**

Large amounts of pre-made vitamin A is found in animal products (meat, eggs, and milk) and supplements, but this form can accumulate in the body and lead to toxicity. The safest way to boost vitamin A levels is to consume more carotenoids. Certain carotenoids can be converted into active vitamin A in the body and this conversion is tightly regulated – you will never develop a vitamin A overload from carotenoid intake.

Useful for:
- **Keratomalacia**

Beta-carotene

Beta-carotene (β-Carotene) is a richly coloured, red-orange pigment found in fruits and vegetables. In its conversion to vitamin A, one molecule of beta-carotene creates two molecules of vitamin A. This is the highest yield of vitamin A from any carotenoid, giving beta-carotene an essential role in preventing diseases that are associated with vitamin A deficiency, such as **keratomalacia**. Beta-carotene is also an antioxidant and has the ability to absorb light within the eye.

CAUTION: In current and former smokers, beta-carotene *supplementation* can increase the risk of lung cancer. Recently, the substitution of beta-carotene with other carotenoids, namely **lutein and zeaxanthin**, has been shown to have a comparably beneficial effect to beta-carotene supplementation. Dietary sources are considered to be completely safe.

Dietary Sources:
- Carrots
- Sweet potato
- Butternut squash
- Green leafy vegetables, such as spinach, kale, broccoli, turnip greens, and Swiss chard
- Melons, such as cantaloupe
- Sour cherries
- Orange fruits, such as mangoes, persimmons, papayas, and apricots

Useful for:
- **General Eye Health**
- **Glaucoma**

Lutein

Lutein is a deep yellow pigment with powerful antioxidant capacities in many areas of the eye. It is sometimes called the 'eye vitamin' (though it isn't a vitamin, and it works throughout the body!). As a major pigment in the **macular pigment**, lutein filters light and protects eye tissues from sunlight, blue light, and UV damage.

Dietary Sources:
- Kale
- Other green leafy vegetables, such as spinach, Swiss chard, mustard greens, turnip greens, watercress, and Brussels sprouts
- Broccoli
- Sweet corn
- Yellow squash and butternut squash
- Kiwi fruit
- Grapes
- Oranges
- Courgettes (zucchini) (Sommerburg, et al., 1998)

Useful for:
- **General Eye Health**
- **Vision Support**
- **Age-Related Macular Degeneration**
- **Cataracts**
- **Glaucoma**

Zeaxanthin

Like lutein, zeaxanthin is a pigment found in the **macular pigment** of the eye. Its name is derived from merging *Zea mays*, the scientific name for yellow corn, and *Xanthos*, the Greek word for yellow. Guess what coloured pigment it provides. You got it – yellow! This pigment absorbs blue light waves and protects the eye against damage. Lutein and zeaxanthin are commonly found together in nature and appear to have a synergistic relationship where they work better together than in isolation.

Dietary Sources:
- Kale
- Dark green leafy vegetables, such as spinach, turnip greens, collard greens, romaine lettuce, mustard greens, and watercress
- Paprika
- Corn
- Saffron
- Spirulina

Useful for:
- **General Eye Health**
- **Vision Support**
- **Age-Related Macular Degeneration**
- **Cataracts**
- **Glaucoma**

Meso-zeaxanthin

Meso-zeaxanthin was discovered much later than lutein and zeaxanthin and, therefore, research is still in comparatively early days. This carotenoid is found in the central retina, along with lutein and zeaxanthin, and they join together to form the **macular pigment**. Each of these three carotenoids absorbs a slightly different wavelength and intensity of blue light to strongly shield the retina against light damage. But when it comes to antioxidant capabilities, meso-zeaxanthin is the clear leader – it has been shown to have almost twice the protective capacity as lutein.

Meso-zeaxanthin is found in the very centre of the macula, while the other two carotenoids are slightly off to the sides. However, zeaxanthin, lutein, and meso-zeaxanthin are always more powerful when combined together.

It's currently unclear whether meso-zeaxanthin is readily available in the human diet, or whether it's created in the body from lutein. Research has found that it is present in the skin and flesh of some fatty fish, but supplementation is recommended to really boost meso-zeaxanthin levels (Nolan, et al., 2013). Note that it is not the same as 'regular' zeaxanthin – meso-zeaxanthin is a different molecular shape and absorbs light wave frequencies that zeaxanthin cannot.

Dietary Sources:
- Trout, sardines, and salmon (with the skin on)
- Possibly egg yolk and corn

Useful for:
- **General Eye Health**
- **Vision Support**
- **Age-Related Macular Degeneration**
- **Cataracts**
- **Glaucoma**

Astaxanthin

Astaxanthin is a red-orange pigment with powerful antioxidant capacity – in fact, it has over 6,000 times the free radical scavenging capacity of **vitamin C**! It has an uncommon ability to pass through the protective blood-ocular barrier in the eye. This barrier prevents most harmful drugs and many nutrients from entering the eyes, but astaxanthin is small enough to pass through the barrier, flowing into the aqueous fluid and retina where it protects the macula and optic nerve against oxidative damage (Hashimoto, et al., 2013; Otsuka, et al., 2013).

In nature, it is found in anything red, but particularly in proteins with a pinkish-orange colour – think seafood and ocean algae!

Dietary Sources:
- Salmon
- Shrimp
- Algae
- Krill

Useful for:
- **General Eye Health**
- **Vision Support**

Lycopene

Lycopene is a bright red pigment that, once ingested, can be found in the retina and blood vessels throughout the eye (Bernstein, et al., 2001). Like other carotenoids, it may help to absorb light waves that could cause **oxidative stress.** It is a powerful antioxidant in its own right, but it can also donate electrons and 'sacrifice' itself to boost levels of lutein and zeaxanthin in the eye.

Fun fact: Too much lycopene can turn your skin orange!

Dietary Sources:
- Cooked tomatoes, including tomato sauce, chutney, and pasta sauce
- Watermelon
- Papaya
- Asparagus
- Parsley
- Sea buckthorn

Useful for:
- **Cataracts**
- **Age-Related Macular Degeneration**

2. B-Group Vitamins

The B-group vitamins perform essential roles within the eye tissues and fluids. They are key coenzymes in cellular energy production, support nerve conduction and signalling between cells, and indirectly protect against **oxidative stress** and inflammation. The trick with B vitamins is that they *must* be taken together – supplementing with one B vitamin alone can throw the rest out of balance.

Vitamin B1 (Thiamine) plays a key role in eye health. As well as playing a role in metabolic pathways to produce cellular energy, thiamine is involved in nervous system stimulation. It modulates the electrical activity between nerves to convey the right message – this is especially useful in the optic nerve where electrical signals from the retina are passed to the brain.

A low level of vitamin B1 is really bad news – **beriberi** is a disease caused by vitamin B1 deficiency and it involves loss of muscle control, involuntary eye movements, double vision, and even hallucinations. Thiamine deficiency is commonly associated with alcohol abuse; alcohol quickly depletes all B vitamins but *especially* thiamine. However, it can also occur as a result of diarrhoea. Serious damage to the optic nerve and vision loss has been observed within just three weeks of thiamine deficiency (Gratton & Lam, 2014).

Dietary Sources:
- Meat
- Salmon
- Legumes (lentils, chickpeas, black beans etc.)
- Grains, cereals, and bread
- Yeast
- Wheat germ
- Soy milk

Vitamin B2 (Riboflavin) is also used to produce cellular energy that keeps eye tissues alive, healthy, and responsive to stimulation. Riboflavin is essential for the metabolism of **vitamin B6** and **folate** and, therefore, plays a role in methylation (see: **Vitamin B6** and **Folate**). It is also needed for protein metabolism to hold together the structures of the eye and for the production of neurotransmitters that influence vision. These brain chemicals include dopamine and serotonin. Riboflavin also supports powerful antioxidants that protect eye tissues against **oxidative stress**.

Dietary Sources:
- Dairy (milk, cheese, yoghurt)
- Eggs
- Green vegetables
- Fruits
- Whole grains

Vitamin B3 (Niacin) is another B vitamin that helps to regenerate the antioxidants in the eye. It can also regenerate **vitamin C** to control **oxidative stress** in the eye tissues. It has a further use as a coenzyme in the metabolism of carbohydrates and can help to reduce the impact of blood sugar dysregulation and **glycation** on eye tissues. It works with **vitamin B2** to metabolise **vitamin B6** and **folate** and, therefore, has a role in **methylation** (see: **Folate**). Deep in the cell, niacin is required for effective DNA synthesis and healthy cell growth.

Dietary Sources:
- Fish and meat
- Whole grains
- Seeds
- Legumes (lentils, chickpeas, black beans, etc.)
- Coffee and tea
- Green vegetables

Note: There is no vitamin B4!

Vitamin B5 (Pantothenic Acid). *Pantos* means 'everywhere' in Greek – an appropriate name, since vitamin B5 is found widely distributed throughout nature. This means that developing a vitamin B5 deficiency is highly unlikely except in cases of total malnutrition and starvation. The name also reflects the fact that it works in conjunction with other nutrients. In fact, its major role is in the metabolism of carbohydrates and proteins to provide cellular energy and structural integrity to the eye.

Dietary Sources:
- Eggs
- Dairy
- Legumes
- Whole grains
- Potatoes
- Mushrooms
- Broccoli
- Avocados
- Small amounts found in all other foods!

Vitamin B6 (Pyridoxine) is actually a group of six similar molecules that are interchangeable. Vitamin B6 is involved in hundreds, if not thousands, of enzymatic reactions throughout the body. It is often the 'go' switch, or the ignition required for the metabolic process to proceed.

Vitamin B6 is involved in blood formation, nerve signalling, producing hormones, and metabolising homocysteine (see: **Folate**).

Dietary Sources:
- Whole grains
- Bananas
- Nuts
- Fortified cereals

Vitamin B7 (Biotin) is required for eye cells to progress normally through their life cycle. A deficiency of biotin will stop cells from being able to multiply and knowing when to self-destruct. It is also required for cellular energy production, the metabolism of amino acids into proteins, and the production of neurotransmitters such as dopamine.

Dietary Sources:
- Soybeans
- Eggs
- Cereals
- Legumes
- Nuts

Note: There is no vitamin B8!

Vitamin B9 (Folate) is involved in a huge range of metabolic processes throughout the body and within the eye. Along with **vitamin B6** and **vitamin B12,** folate is an essential component of the **methylation cycle.** This cycle takes homocysteine (a pro-inflammatory amino acid) and metabolises it into anti-inflammatory metabolites *OR* regenerates it into another amino acid, methionine. These cycles can't operate without adequate amounts of **folate, vitamin B12,** and **vitamin B6.**

With low levels of these B vitamins, homocysteine levels can stack up in the body. High levels of homocysteine have been linked to diseases of the cardiovascular system (which includes the small blood vessels that supply eye tissues with oxygen and nutrients). Recent research suggests that homocysteine levels also have a correlation with major eye diseases, including **glaucoma** and **cataracts.**

Folate is also an essential ingredient in the development of red and white blood cells. Red blood cells are necessary for healthy eyes – without an adequate supply of the oxygen that they carry, eye tissues cannot function and die off. White blood cells provide immune support against a wide range of pathogens that can infect the eyes. In this way, folate can protect the eyes against **conjunctivitis** and **blepharitis.**

Dietary Sources:
- Mushrooms
- Green vegetables (especially spinach, Brussels sprouts, asparagus, broccoli, and turnip greens)
- Peanuts
- Legumes (especially pinto beans, black beans, and lentils)
- Fruits (especially oranges and strawberries)
- Fortified flours and grains

No vitamin B10 or B11, either!

Vitamin B12 (Cobalamin) works closely with **folate** in the metabolism of homocysteine and in the production of red and white blood cells. It is essential for protecting the small blood vessels that supply the eye tissues with oxygen and nutrients.

Vitamin B12 is required for the maintenance of the strength and integrity of myelin, a protective sheeting that covers the optic nerve and other nerve fibres in the eye. A deficiency will slowly eat away at the myelin, causing poor nerve conduction and eventual nerve destruction.

There are two problems with vitamin B12 – it is *only* found in large quantities in very few foods, and its absorption in the intestines is very complex. Consequently, a deficiency is very common in older people. There seems to be a correlation between vitamin B12 and many age-related eye conditions, such as **cataracts** and **age-related macular degeneration.**

Dietary Sources:
- Meat
- Fish
- Eggs
- Dairy
- Fortified cereals and grains
- Small amounts found in legumes, mushrooms, and some yeasts

3. Vitamin C

Vitamin C, also known as ascorbic acid, has a relatively uncomplicated chemical structure but very complex role in the body tissues. Vitamin C is required for the synthesis of collagen (a flexible connective tissue that forms most of the eye's structure), the creation of neurotransmitters (nervous system and brain chemicals) that control the focussing of the lens, and antioxidant activities that protect eye tissues against **oxidative damage**. Vitamin C actually *reverses* oxidation by donating electrons and hydrogen ions. It is also a direct free radical scavenger and regenerates other antioxidants, such as **vitamin E** and glutathione.

Dietary Sources:
- Kiwi fruit
- Strawberries
- Red capsicum (red peppers)
- Asparagus
- Papaya
- Cantaloupe
- Cauliflower
- Citrus fruits, such as oranges

Useful for:
- **General Eye Health**

- **Cataracts**
- **Age-Related Macular Degeneration**

4. Vitamin D

Vitamin D is actually more of a hormone than a vitamin. In fact, it is created from a steroid hormone and works closely with the endocrine (hormone-related) system throughout the body. The hundreds of roles that vitamin D exhibits in the body can be grouped into two categories – roles where it regulates gene expression and roles where it activates cellular signals.

Within the eye, vitamin D has been shown to protect against a number of eye diseases through these two main roles. It enhances the immune defences and healthy cell proliferation in the cornea, lens, ciliary body, macular pigment, and retina. It also activates cellular signalling so that eye cells can clearly communicate what they need for their health (Reins & McDermott, 2015).

Most of the body's vitamin D is produced during a chemical reaction between the sun and the skin. Cells in the top layers of the skin interact with UV-B rays from sunlight to create pre-vitamin D. Pre-vitamin D is then released into the bloodstream and activated through the kidneys and liver with the help of other nutrient co-factors including **magnesium** and **B vitamins.** Through these reactions, pre-vitamin D is transformed into its bioactive form – vitamin D3. It is suspected that the eyes may also be a site of this activation (Reins & McDermott, 2015).

Despite the abundance of sunlight available in most parts of the world, vitamin D deficiency is incredibly common, with an estimated one billion people worldwide currently suffering from low levels. Taking a supplement and increasing dietary sources can help to boost vitamin D stores.

Dietary Sources:
- Fatty Fish
- Beef
- Liver
- Eggs

- Mushrooms exposed to sunlight

Useful for:
- **Vision Support**
- **General Eye Health**

5. Vitamin E

Vitamin E is a fat-soluble antioxidant that has the unique ability to protect against free radical attacks in the fatty environments of cellular membranes, nerve coverings, and in the fibres of the eye's lens. 'Vitamin E' actually refers to eight very similar compounds called tocopherols and tocotrienols.

The primary function of vitamin E is its antioxidant action which directly quenches free radicals, protects against lipid peroxidation (oxidative degradation of lipids), and regenerates **vitamin C** and glutathione. It also functions as a cell-signalling molecule and influences how quickly cells regenerate. Vitamin E is essential for the function and health of all eye tissues.

Dietary Sources:
- Wheat germ
- Sunflower seeds
- Soybeans
- Peanuts
- Cashews
- Hazelnuts
- Almonds
- Whole-grain cereals
- Green vegetables

Useful for:
- **Cataracts**
- **Glaucoma**
- **Age-Related Macular Degeneration**

6. Magnesium

Magnesium is an essential mineral and electrolyte. Over 60% of the magnesium in the body is found in the skeletal system, but the remaining 40% is used in essential physiological reactions. Magnesium is a key co-factor in enzymatic reactions that create cellular energy, replicate DNA, create new proteins, control blood glucose levels, and protect against **hyperglycaemia**. It is known as a 'relaxing' nutrient – it helps muscles to relax and blood vessels to dilate. Magnesium is quickly excreted from the body during times of stress, illness, or exercise but is usually easily replenished by taking a supplement or eating more magnesium-rich foods.

Dietary Sources:
- Nuts
- Legumes
- Whole-grain cereals (especially oats and barley)
- Beans (especially pinto, kidney and haricot (navy) beans)
- Peanut butter
- Green vegetables
- Spices

Useful for:
- **Glaucoma**

7. Sodium

Sodium doesn't just make table salt – it is also an essential electrolyte found mostly in the body's extracellular fluid, nerve tissues, and muscle cells. However, the average western diet contains so much sodium that it can result in a build-up in the body and cause issues throughout the **microcirculation**, particularly in the blood vessels of the eyes.

As a major electrolyte, sodium is required in adequate amounts to **balance electrolytes** within the eye. Too much sodium has been associated with hypertension (high blood pressure), which can increase the pressure inside the eye and may contribute to diseases such as **age-related macular degeneration** and **glaucoma**.

Dietary Sources:
- Celery
- Carrots
- Spinach
- Beetroot
- Milk

High Sodium Dietary Sources:
- Refined carbohydrate foods (e.g. bread, pizza, pasta)
- Cheese
- Snack foods (e.g. crisps, pretzels, popcorn)
- Soft drinks
- Processed meats (e.g. ham, pepperoni)
- Boxed cereals
- Cakes and pies

Caution for:
- **Cataracts**
- **Age-Related Macular Degeneration**
- **Glaucoma**

8. Zinc

Zinc is a trace nutrient that is involved in hundreds of enzymatic reactions throughout the body. It has four major functions in the eye: it protects against **oxidative damage** as a major component of antioxidant enzymes called **superoxide dismutase (SOD)** and **nitric oxide synthase (NOS);** it protects against eye infections by participating in immune reactions; it supports the growth and proliferation of healthy cells by participating in DNA replication; and it gives tissues their strength and integrity as part of zinc fingers.

Zinc fingers are finger-like loops that give proteins their structure and strength. Without zinc, the structures of the eyes (and the whole body) would be a wobbly mess!

Zinc is also an essential part of insulin, a hormone that transports sugar out of the blood and into cells. A 2012 systematic review and meta-analysis of 22 studies demonstrated that zinc supplementation can reduce the level of glucose in the blood, control **hyperglycaemia**, and protect against damage in the eye caused by **glycation** (Jayawardena, et al., 2012).

Dietary Sources:
- Meat
- Dairy products
- Whole grains (especially bran and germ)
- Leafy vegetables
- Root vegetables

Useful for:
- **General Eye Health**
- **Vision Support**
- **Age-Related Macular Degeneration**

9. Omega-3 Essential Fatty Acids

Essential fatty acids are small to medium fat molecules. The human body cannot efficiently produce its own essential fatty acids, so they must be included in the diet. There are two major types – omega-3 and omega-6. All essential fatty acids participate in the regulation of inflammation throughout the body, but their metabolism can create either pro-inflammatory or anti-inflammatory chemical messengers. Omega-3 essential fatty acids are considered 'anti-inflammatory' because their metabolism creates chemicals that block the inflammatory signals from other fats. This can help to reduce **oxidative stress.** Omega-3 intake is also associated with flexible cellular membranes – these allow substances to flow in and out of the cell as needed and help cells to communicate with each other.

The three main omega-3 fatty acids are alpha-linolenic acid (ALA), eicosapentaenoic acid (EPA) and docosahexaenoic acid (DHA). EPA and DHA are more useful in the human body. ALA can be converted into EPA and DHA in the liver, but the process is inefficient so it can be difficult to get enough EPA and DHA by consuming sources of ALA alone.

Increasing your dietary intake of omega-3 is one way to reduce inflammation. Another is to reduce the intake of other pro-inflammatory fats, such as excessive omega-6 essential fatty acids. The ideal ratio of omega-6 to omega-3 essential fatty acids is 2-3:1. In the standard western diet, however, the ratio tends to be 15:1. This high omega-6 ratio has been associated with cardiovascular disease, inflammatory conditions, and autoimmune issues (Simopoulus, 2002). Omega-6 is found in meat, sunflower oil, corn oil, soybean oil, cottonseed oil, and canola oil – avoid these and opt for omega-3-rich foods and oils to rebalance your omega-6 to omega-3 ratio!

Dietary Sources of DHA & EPA:
- Fatty fish, such as salmon and sardines

Dietary Sources of ALA:
- Walnuts
- Olive oil
- Chia seeds
- Hemp seeds
- Flax seeds

Useful for:
- **General Eye Health**
- **Dry Eye Syndrome**
- **Blepharitis**

10. Omega-7 Fatty Acids

Unlike omega-3, omega-7 fatty acids are non-essential; the human body can make its own omega-7 from other fats. Recent research, however, has found that this fatty acid may have therapeutic benefits when taken in supplemental form. It has potent antibacterial, anti-inflammatory, and soothing actions on the eyes and it could help to control **hyperglycaemia** and **oxidative stress** (de Souza, et al., 2018).

Dietary Sources:
- Sea buckthorn berries
- Milk
- Yoghurt

- Cheese
- Macadamia nuts

Useful for:
- **Dry Eye Syndrome**
- **Conjunctivitis**

11. Carbohydrates

Carbohydrates are the major source of energy fuel in the human diet and they supply half or more of our total daily calories. Carbohydrates are either polysaccharides, such as starches from cereal grains and vegetables; or simple sugars, such as sucrose, lactose, and fructose. Almost all carbohydrates are broken down into small sugar molecules during digestion. These small molecules (called glucose) are then used throughout the body to create cellular energy (with the help of co-factors such as **B-group vitamins** and **magnesium**).

Normally, the level of sugars found in circulation (blood sugar levels) is regulated tightly within a narrow range by hormones such as insulin. Certain health conditions and dietary patterns can disrupt this regulation, resulting in high blood sugar (**hyperglycaemia**).

Generally speaking, refined carbohydrates are more likely to cause a spike in blood glucose, while whole foods with high fibre content can help to keep sugar levels stable. People with diagnosed insulin resistance, diabetes, or other glycaemic conditions should seek personalised advice from a qualified nutritionist or dietitian before making any dietary changes.

Dietary Sources:
- Whole grains (e.g. brown rice, barley, buckwheat)
- Fruits and vegetables
- Nuts and seeds
- Legumes (e.g. lentils, chickpeas, haricot (navy) beans)
- Popcorn
- Dairy products (no sugar added)

Refined Carbohydrate Dietary Sources:
- White flour and products (e.g. white bread, cakes, etc.)
- Soft drinks and energy drinks
- Alcohol
- Sweets and chocolate bars
- Potato crisps and fries
- Fried foods
- Boxed cereals
- Sugar added to any food (check the ingredients label!)

Caution for:
- **Cataracts**
- **Age-Related Macular Degeneration**

12. Quercetin

Quercetin is a flavonoid pigment found in plants and herbs. It is a potent antioxidant with a high affinity for eye tissues where it protects against **oxidative stress** and tissue damage. Quercetin also interacts with the immune system, where it can strengthen white blood cells against allergy reactions, and it even has antibacterial and antiviral properties.

Dietary Sources:
- Apples
- Onions
- Berries (especially blackberries, blueberries, and raspberries)
- Capers
- Plums
- Kale
- Asparagus
- Broccoli

Useful for:
- **Conjunctivitis**

4. HERBS FOR EYE HEALTH

1. Bilberry
2. Eyebright
3. Goldenseal
4. Tea Tree
5. Turmeric

1. Bilberry (*Vaccinium myrtillus*)

Vaccinium myrtillus is a species of the bilberry family that is used as a go-to in herbal medicine for relieving eye strain and supporting vision. The leaf of the bilberry plant is rich in powerful herbal chemicals that are useful for controlling metabolic disorders, such as diabetes, but it is the dark purple fruit that is packed full of eye-loving antioxidants, like anthocyanins, flavonoids, **quercetin**, and **vitamin C.** The pigments in bilberries are so rich that you have to be careful when eating them fresh– the purple colour can stain your skin and clothing!

Along with this powerful antioxidant capacity, bilberry extract has been shown to have antimicrobial actions and can help to repair DNA, strengthen blood vessels in the eyes, regulate gene expression, and control cell growth (Chu, et al., 2011).

Cautions & Side Effects
Bilberry is classified as a Class 1 herb in the USA, indicating that it is safe to consume and there are no reported contraindications to

its use.

However, anthocyanins are powerful antiplatelet agents – this means that they help to stop the blood from clotting and can, therefore, increase the risk of bleeding. Speak to a qualified herbalist or pharmacist before taking bilberry supplements if you also take blood-thinning medications (including aspirin), or are diabetic, pregnant, or breastfeeding.

Stop taking bilberry at least two weeks before any type of surgery and inform your medical team of all supplements and herbal medicines you have taken in the last three months.

Useful for:
   - **General Eye Health**
   - **Cataracts**
   - **Night Vision**

2. Eyebright (*Euphrasia officinalis*)

Eyebright, or *Euphrasia officinalis*, has been used in traditional herbal medicine as an eye tonic for hundreds of years – the name says it all! It is native to Europe but has been successfully introduced to regions throughout the world and now grows throughout Asia and North America. The plant itself is semi-parasitic in that it attaches itself to the roots of other plants and obtains much of its nutrition by 'leeching' nutrients from its host. Every part of the plant, from the ground up, is used in the creation of herbal medicines – stem, leaves, and flowers.

Eyebright is rich in **vitamin C**, **vitamin A**, and essential oils. It has been used since the Middle Ages as a cure for **conjunctivitis** and bloodshot eyes and to relieve inflammation of the lids associated with **blepharitis**.

When it comes to taking it as a herbal medicine, the effects of eyebright depend not only on the quality of the herb itself but also on the solvent used to extract the plant's medicinal constituents. An *in vitro* study from 2014 compared three different types of solvents commonly used in products with eyebright extracts – heptane, ethanol, and ethyl acetate. All three extracts stopped the cells in the cornea from producing pro-inflammatory chemical messengers, but the heptane extracts showed toxic effects on the epithelial cells there (Paduch, et al., 2014).

CAUTION: Beware of heptane extracts! Most commercial eye drops use an ethanol base, but always check the ingredients or speak to a qualified herbalist or naturopath for personalised advice.

Cautions & Side Effects
Allergic reactions are **rare** but possible. Seek IMMEDIATE medical attention if you experience any of these symptoms after taking eyebright:

- Difficulty breathing
- Closing of your throat
- Swelling of your lips, tongue, or face
- Hives

Seek medical attention if you experience other possible side effects:

- A sensation of pressure in the eyes causing tearing, itching, redness, or swelling
- Sensitivity to light
- Vision problems
- Sneezing or runny nose
- A headache that lasts over two hours or does not improve after taking painkillers

Useful for:
- **Blepharitis**
- **Conjunctivitis**

3. Goldenseal (*Hydrastis canadensis*)

Hydrastis canadensis, or goldenseal, is a native North American herb and is part of the buttercup family. It is also known as 'eye balm' or 'eye root', which is a clear hint of what it has been traditionally used for – eye health! Certain Native American tribes used goldenseal as a topical eyewash to treat inflammatory conditions, such as **blepharitis.** However, recent research into the efficacy and safety of goldenseal for the treatment of eye conditions is significantly lacking. We are including it here as an acknowledgement of its traditional use and to recommend caution when self-prescribing.

Cautions & Side Effects

The major active chemical in goldenseal is called berberine and has been shown to stimulate phototoxic effects when applied topically to cells of the eye's lens. This means that using goldenseal eye drops and then exposing the eyes to light (especially sunlight) could cause permanent damage. Only use goldenseal eye drops under the direction and supervision of a qualified herbalist or suitably qualified healthcare professional (Chignell, et al., 2007).

When taken orally, goldenseal can also cause a lot of grief. Taking high doses of berberine can block receptors on certain muscles cells, including cells of the heart, which can exacerbate existing heart conditions – this could be fatal in some cases.

Other possible side effects of low or moderate doses of goldenseal include:
  • Gastrointestinal discomfort
  • Bloating
  • Nervousness
  • Depression
  • Nausea and vomiting
  • Stomach cramps
  • Rapid heartbeat

High doses can lead to paralysis, breathing problems and, potentially, death.

Long-term use of low-to-moderate doses of goldenseal can cause hallucinations and delirium. It can also block the uptake of essential nutrients and lead to a deficiency in **B vitamins**.

CAUTION: Speak to your doctor or pharmacist before taking goldenseal if you are taking any other medicines. Goldenseal stops the liver from processing certain medicines (inhibits cytochrome P450 enzymes) and can, therefore, cause increased side effects or even a potentially fatal toxicity (Etheridge, et al., 2007; Gurley, et al., 2008a; Gurley, et al., 2008b).

Possibly useful for:
- **Blepharitis**
- **Conjunctivitis**

Use with caution!

4. Tea Tree (*Melalueca*)

Tea tree is a native Australian paperbark tree with narrow leaves that are rich in essential oil. This oil is toxic when taken orally, but it is used topically in low concentrations for a variety of skin, hair, and nail conditions. Tea tree oil contains over 98 compounds. It is rich in naturally occurring terpinene, which gives it a powerful antimicrobial action that can eradicate bacteria, viruses, and mites.

Cautions & Side Effects

Tea tree oil is powerful and can cause irritation when applied topically.

Tea tree oil is HIGHLY TOXIC when taken orally and can lead to muscle paralysis. Do NOT drink or consume tea tree oil in any form.

Possible side effects of topical use include:
- Local irritation, such as redness and burning
- Allergic skin rash, such as dermatitis
- Itching
- Stinging

Spot test a small amount of diluted tea tree oil on a small patch of skin at least 48 hours before use to check for allergic reactions.

Always dilute tea tree oil with a carrier oil (such as coconut oil or olive oil) in a 1:3 ratio before use (one drop of tea tree oil to three drops of oil) and use on CLOSED eyes only. Use a weaker dilution if you experience any stinging or burning sensations.

Useful for:
   · **Blepharitis**

5. Turmeric (*Curcuma longa*)

Turmeric (*Curcuma longa*) is a deep yellow-orange culinary spice and herbal medicine from the Indian subcontinent and Southeast Asia. The rhizome of the plant is harvested and used fresh or dried and ground into a fine powder. It has a long history of use in traditional herbal medicine, including Ayurveda and Traditional Chinese Medicine, where it is used in the management of inflammatory conditions, metabolic syndrome, arthritis, and degenerative eye conditions.

Turmeric contains carbohydrates, proteins, and a group of active ingredients called **curcuminoids**. One of these is **curcumin**, the most widely recognised and utilised turmeric compound. It has powerful anti-inflammatory actions in the body and has been traditionally used to maintain the shape and structure of the eyes and to treat **conjunctivitis.**

Most studies on the effects of turmeric use **curcumin extract** and give doses of at least 1g per day. Turmeric itself contains only about 3% curcumin. Therein lies the issue – while including turmeric in the diet may help to maintain general health, a highly concentrated curcumin extract is the only way to benefit from the therapeutic potential found in the latest research.

NOTE: Curcumin is only absorbed when taken with a source of fat and it works better when taken alongside black pepper. The fat brings the curcumin into the intestinal cells, and the piperine from the peppercorns stops the liver from metabolising the curcumin too quickly, keeping it active in the body for longer.

Cautions & Side Effects
The first thing to be aware of when handling turmeric is that it will stain *everything* it touches – but only for 48-72 hours. The bright orange pigments in turmeric are photosensitive and slowly fade away from light exposure.

Turmeric and curcumin extracts are generally considered safe

and do not usually cause side effects. Very high doses may cause:
- Stomach upsets
- Dizziness
- Nausea and diarrhoea
- Bloating
- Acid reflux
- Hypotension (low blood pressure)
- Increased menstrual flow
- Uterine contractions in pregnant women

Speak to a qualified herbalist or naturopath for personalised advice before taking curcumin extracts or turmeric supplements if you:
- Are diabetic
- Are, could be, or are planning to become pregnant
- Suffer from a hormone-related condition (e.g. breast cancer, endometriosis)
- Have, or suspect you may have, an iron deficiency
- Have surgery scheduled

As an anti-clotting agent, turmeric can increase the risk of bleeding. Before taking turmeric, consult your doctor or pharmacist if you're taking blood-thinning medication (anticoagulants). Stop taking turmeric at least two weeks before any type of surgery and inform your medical team of all supplements and herbal medicines you have taken in the last three months.

Useful for:
- **Dry Eye Syndrome**
- **Conjunctivitis**
- **Cataracts**
- **Glaucoma**

5. EYE HEALTH & DISEASE

1. General Eye Health
2. Vision Support
3. Age-Related Macular Degeneration
4. Dry Eyes
5. Cataracts
6. Glaucoma
7. Night Blindness (Nyctalopia)
8. Keratomalacia
9. Blepharitis
10. Conjunctivitis

1. General Eye Health

The eye, like all organs of the body, strives to maintain homeostasis – a stable, predictable state. Key nutrients support the physical structures of the eye while others promote healthy physiological processes, such as cellular division, clearing out old and damaged cells, encouraging the flow of aqueous humour, and protecting the eye against infections.

Carotenoids

Beta-Carotene

Beta-carotene is an antioxidant carotenoid. After it goes through extensive metabolism within the liver, beta-carotene yields the most vitamin A of all the carotenoids. This is a key role for beta-carotene and can usually supply enough vitamin A to meet the body's physiological needs. Because of this potential to convert into vitamin A, beta-carotene is essential for basic eye health – it is required for the absorption of light in the retina and for the prevention of diseases of deficiency, such as **keratomalacia.** Beta-carotene is also directly involved in controlling the life-and-death cycles of eye cells – it helps to control cell division and programmed cell death.

Lutein

Although lutein can't be converted into vitamin A, it is still an essential carotenoid in eye health. In terms of concentration, lutein (along with zeaxanthin and meso-zeaxanthin) is more present in the retina than in any other tissue in the body. The highest concentration is found in the macular pigment, where it selectively absorbs blue light. Blue light causes a hundred times more light-induced damage to the eye than orange light. As a result of its selective filtering capabilities, lutein can prevent permanent damage to photoreceptors in the retina (Koushan, et al., 2013). Lutein is also directly involved in quenching free radicals and controlling the level of **oxidative stress** in the eye.

Zeaxanthin

Zeaxanthin is often found alongside lutein and meso-zeaxanthin and these three carotenoids have similar roles within the eye. Zeaxanthin also has a light-absorbing capacity in the macular pigment, but its major role is in programmed cell death. It is able to stop the death of cells that are still needed by the body while simultaneously allowing dangerous or damaged cells to die off (Demmig-Adams & Adams, 2013). People who have higher levels of this carotenoid in their bodies are more likely to have better general eye health and a lower risk of developing eye-related cancers (Tanaka, et al., 2012).

Astaxanthin

Astaxanthin is a red-orange coloured carotenoid and a strong antioxidant. Several studies have shown that it is a powerful protector against oxidative stress in the retina and against chemical messengers that create inflammation. In both animal and human studies, astaxanthin supplementation has been shown to be most effective when combined with lutein. Together, they can protect all eye tissues and the aqueous humour against **oxidative stress** (Yeh, et al., 2016).

A 2013 study sought to find out if taking an astaxanthin supplement had any real impact on the levels of this carotenoid inside the eye and whether it really did help with oxidative stress levels. The researchers recruited 35 patients who were undergoing bilateral cataract surgery. During the surgery on the first eye, surgeons took a sample of aqueous humour from within the eye. The participants were then instructed to take 6mg of astaxanthin each day for two weeks. More aqueous humour was taken during the following surgery on the other eye, and the humour was compared to the original sample. After two weeks of astaxanthin supplementation, there was a significant increase in antioxidant activity within the second aqueous humour – specifically, superoxide enzyme activity was markedly raised while the level of total **oxidative stress** and free radicals was significantly lowered. This shows that even two weeks of astaxanthin supplementation can promote eye health and protect all of the eye tissues and aqueous humour against **oxidative damage** (Hashimoto, et al., 2013).

Vitamin C

Vitamin C is a powerful antioxidant that has the capacity to regenerate or 'recycle' other antioxidants throughout the body. In the eye, vitamin C is an important co-factor in the formation of collagen, a connective tissue that is present in the highest amounts in the cornea. It also promotes the health of the blood vessels that supply the eyes and enhances the function of nerve cells in the retina. The immune system requires a large amount of vitamin C to protect the eye against pathogen infections and, as a potent antioxidant, this key nutrient can prevent **oxidative stress** that leads to tissue damage and many eye diseases (Chambial, et al., 2013).

Vitamin D

Vitamin D is the 'sunshine vitamin', created from UV-B radiation. It acts more like a hormone than a vitamin and is sometimes talked of as a 'prohormone' that is essential for health throughout the entire body.

Vitamin D has roles in immune function, the regulation of insulin and blood glucose levels, tissue structure, the regulation of inflammation, DNA synthesis, and cell proliferation. In the eyes, vitamin D is concentrated in the lens, aqueous humour, tear film, cornea, ciliary body, and retina.

Deficiency of this prohormone has been linked to an increased risk of **age-related macular degeneration** and diabetic retinopathy (Richer & Pizzimenti, 2013).

Zinc

Zinc is an essential trace mineral involved in maintaining the health of the retina. It also influences all facets of metabolism within the eye. Zinc has key roles in antioxidant and immune functions, and in the structure and protection of proteins and cell membranes. The Age-Related Eye Disease Study (AREDS) found that zinc was needed at a level well above the recommended daily allowance to reduce the risk of developing advanced age-related macular degeneration (AMD, or sometimes ARMD) by up to 25% (Age-Related Eye Disease Study Research Group, 2001; Rasmussen, et al., 2013).

Omega-3

Omega-3 essential fatty acids have a number of actions that may provide protection to the nerves of the retina. Within the eye, omega-3s are involved in influencing certain metabolic processes that affect **oxidative stress** levels, inflammation, and blood supply via **microcirculation**.

Eicosapentaenoic acid (EPA) is an omega-3 fatty acid that is found in dense concentration in the eyes. It is a powerful anti-inflammatory agent. The metabolism of EPA reduces inflammation throughout the body in two ways: it produces anti-inflammatory chemical messengers, and it blocks other fats from producing pro-inflammatory agents and oxidative stress.

Docosahexaenoic Acid (DHA) is another long-chain fatty acid. It is created from EPA through a metabolic process that requires **vitamin B1** (thiamine) as a co-factor. DHA is even more important for eye health than EPA. As well as keeping inflammation down, it is found in large amounts in the retina where it affects retinal cell-signalling – the way that cells communicate with each other. DHA is essential for a process called 'phototransduction'. This is where light is converted into electrical signals that are then passed down the optic nerve to be interpreted by the brain. Essentially, it is required for vision to work properly (Rasmussen, et al., 2013).

Both DHA and EPA protect the tissues of the circulatory system against oxidative stress, ensuring that adequate supplies of blood and nutrients reach the small and delicate blood vessels throughout the eyes.

2. Vision Support

Normal Vision

In normal vision, light rays enter through the lens and are focussed on to the retina by the cornea. The ciliary muscles adjust the shape of the lens to properly focus the images. This creates a sharp image that is then transmitted to the brain via the optic nerve. Vision issues, like short-sightedness or long-sightedness, also known as **refractive errors**, occur when the eye is unable to focus images sharply on the retina, resulting in blurred vision.

Myopia (Short-Sightedness)

Myopia can occur when the eye grows too long from front-to-back (this is also known as the **axial length**). This extension of length creates issues with focussing, or a 'refractive error'. Where images are normally focussed sharply onto the retina, the extra space between the lens and the retina now means that the 'focus' of the light hits a spot *before* the retina. Consequently, myopia results in distant images appearing blurred while up-close detail can be seen clearly.

Myopia is traditionally considered an unsolvable medical problem; while it can be corrected with glasses, contact lenses, or surgery, it can never be 'cured'. Part of the issue is that the medical world doesn't yet understand all of the causes and underlying mechanisms that lead to changes in the axial length of the eye. Without knowing the cause, it is impossible to find a permanent and complete prevention of, or treatment for, myopia. Recent research has found some hints, though. **Oxidative stress** appears to be a core underlying cause of the structural changes that lead to myopia. Free radicals can damage the retina and lens tissues and interfere with basic metabolic processes within the eye. This kind of oxidative damage occurs when the available antioxidants in the eye tissues are overwhelmed by a high level of oxidative stress (Francisco, et al., 2015).

Hyperopia (Far-Sightedness)

In hyperopia, either the curve of the cornea is too flat or the axial length of the eye is too short. This causes light waves to reach the retina *before* the point of focus which results in the point of focus forming *after* the retina. In adults, both near and far objects will appear blurred. Children generally only experience mild blurred vision, as they have more flexible lenses which are more able to move to accommodate the hyperopia. Again, **oxidative stress** may play a role in the development of this common vision issue.

Astigmatism

Astigmatism refers to a problem with the curvature of the cornea. Ideally, the entire curve of the cornea is symmetrical. With astigmatism, certain parts of the cornea are flatter or more curved, resulting in a non-spherical shape. When light hits a cornea with astigmatism, the rays focus on different points in the retina, causing blurred vision at any distance. Most people have a certain level of astigmatism.

Floaters

Floaters are small spots that drift through your field of vision – they can look like black or grey specks, cobwebs, or spots. When you look directly at them, they tend to dart away out of your direct vision. At best, floaters are a barely noticeable – at worst, they become a visual distraction. This is a very common condition called 'miodesopsia' and research suggests floaters may be more common in people who are short- or far-sighted than those with normal vision (Webb, et al., 2013).

Collagen and other tissues naturally break down and float in the aqueous fluid within the eye. When these small pieces of tissue float between the retina and the lens, they appear in the vision. They look like 'floaters' because they are literally floating in the aqueous fluid! Anything that increases the breakdown of tissues can cause floaters, including **oxidative stress**, UV damage, inflammation, diabetes, and free radicals.

Lutein, Zeaxanthin & Meso-Zeaxanthin

Lutein is a powerful antioxidant. With the link between myopia and oxidative stress, lutein may help to protect against tissue changes that lead to axial lengthening and blurred vision. It can reduce inflammation and promote healthy structural changes to the retina and the nerves in the eyes. A 2017 study that initially investigated vitamin D accidentally identified a link between high levels of lutein and a lower risk of myopia (Williams, et al., 2017). The participants who had the highest levels of lutein concentrations had a 40% reduction in odds of developing myopia.

Lutein, zeaxanthin, and meso-zeaxanthin together make up the **macular pigment**. This layer of nutrients catches blue light waves and protects the retina against oxidative damage. In one study, participants who took a nutritional supplement that contained 10mg of lutein, 2mg zeaxanthin, and 10mg of meso-zeaxanthin experienced improvements to their vision (Loughman, et al., 2012). Specifically, these nutrients may help to reduce glare and halos and improve the contrast between light and dark.

These three carotenoids may also help to reduce floaters. By working their antioxidant actions throughout the eye, they can reduce the breakdown of collagen and other eye tissues (Hu, et al., 2011).

Astaxanthin

A 2002 study found that taking 5mg of astaxanthin for four weeks could improve the vision of people who work at computer screens. The astaxanthin appeared to improve the lens accommodation to better focus on nearby objects and also helped to counteract mild blurring from hyperopia and eye fatigue (Nagaki, et al., 2002).

A later study that used a higher dose of astaxanthin found an even greater improvement in vision measurements. Twenty-two middle-aged and older people with eye strain symptoms were recruited and given 6mg of astaxanthin each day for four weeks. The researchers assessed signs of myopia and hyperopia before and after the supplementation. Sure enough, measurements of lens accommodation were significantly improved. Participants also reported that their symptoms had improved and felt they had sharper vision (Kajita, et al., 2009).

Astaxanthin appears to work synergistically with other eye-supporting nutrients and herbs. A 2014 study found that taking a formulation of 4mg of astaxanthin with 10mg of lutein, 20mg of bilberry, and 50mg of DHA for four weeks could significantly improve symptoms of eye fatigue, vision, and measurements of lens accommodation (Kono, et al., 2014).

Vitamin D

Myopia has recently been linked to time spent outdoors (or lack thereof). Children with short-sightedness tend to spend less time outdoors than those with non-myopic vision. This is not just a coincidence, and neither is preferring to spend time indoors a symptom of having poor vision – it appears that indoor time can actually increase the risk of developing myopia (Mutti, et al., 2002).

Theories suggest that frequently resting the eyes on objects that are further away while outdoors may help to train to eyes to retain long-distance focus, but it may have more to do with sun exposure. Sunlight stimulates the release of **dopamine** in the retina. Dopamine is a neurotransmitter or 'nervous system chemical' that has been shown to stop abnormal growth in axial length. Sunlight is also a precursor for **vitamin D** and a 2011 study found that teens and young adults with myopia had correspondingly low levels of vitamin D (Mutti & Marks, 2011). With its various roles in DNA synthesis and growth regulation, it is likely that having healthy levels of vitamin D could protect against cell changes that lead to the stretching of axial length.

A larger 2016 study confirmed these findings and identified a significant connection between low outdoor exposure, low vitamin D levels, and extended axial length (Tideman, et al., 2016). If outdoor time isn't available to you, vitamin D supplementation may help to prevent the progression of myopia.

Zinc

Zinc is required for the replication of cells in all tissues in the human body and it is a co-factor in superoxide dismutase (SOD) and nitric oxide synthase (NOS), powerful antioxidant enzymes. Because of this, it could help to protect the eye against any axial lengthening or shortening that leads to vision problems. Animal studies have shown that zinc supplementation can prevent the elongation of the axial length. It can also strengthen the power of light reflected from the lens and retina, which can improve vision in myopia (Huibi, et al., 2001).

Zinc is required for the proper formation of tissues throughout the eye. It gives strength to tissues like collagen, so it could also help to prevent floaters.

However, the relationship between zinc and other trace minerals is just as important as the total level of zinc in circulation. An early study in 1990 investigated the link between zinc levels and tissue changes in the retina of myopic eyes. The study found that *high* levels of zinc with correspondingly *low* levels of copper was associated with a quicker progression of short-sightedness (Silverstone, 1990). Zinc and copper work together throughout the body, but this working relationship is created by *competing* with each other; when either copper or zinc are found in high amounts, the other will be low. Low levels of copper can also cause issues with the shape of the eyes. A balance of both zinc and copper is needed.

High levels of zinc can compromise copper levels. Zinc and copper are stored inside cells by the same 'carrier'. When in storage, both minerals are rendered immobile and inactive. High levels of zinc in the general circulation *or* in the gastrointestinal tract stimulate the creation of more of these carriers. Copper can become trapped in the gastrointestinal tract by these excess carriers and never make it into general circulation. In this way, high levels of zinc can create a copper deficiency (Fischer, et al., 1981; Hoffman, et al., 1988; Wapnir & Balkman, 1991).

Because of this, long-term or high-dose zinc supplementation can throw copper out of balance and effectively undo any benefit that zinc supplementation had in the first place. To safely boost your zinc levels and maintain copper equilibrium, take less than 30mg of supplemental zinc per day and keep an eye on your copper levels, especially if you are taking zinc supplements for longer than three months.

Bilberry

Bilberry is rich in powerful antioxidant nutrients that can combat any underlying oxidative stress in myopia. Specifically, the anthocyanins found in bilberry have been shown to accelerate the repair of eye tissues (Kamiya, et al., 2013). Animal studies show that bilberry extract can protect the eye against structural changes and could be a useful treatment in preventing the progression of myopia (Deng, et al., 2016).

A 2013 prospective study examined the effects of fermented bilberry extracts on people with myopia. The placebo-controlled trial involved 30 participants with myopia who were randomly assigned to one of two groups. The first group was given 400mg of fermented bilberry extract each day while the second group was given a placebo. After four weeks, participants who took the bilberry extract showed significant improvements in how well their eyes detected contrast sensitivity (an important aspect of vision that helps us to see in low light or environments with fog or glare). Driving at night requires excellent contrast sensitivity and is, therefore, one of the first activities that becomes difficult to do with myopia. The bilberry group also experienced a subjective improvement in lens accommodation – the people who took the herbal extract felt that it was easier to quickly focus on objects at different distances. The researchers used fermented bilberry extract as previous evidence had shown that the fermentation process creates a new and unique compound with health-promoting properties, but it is likely that standard bilberry would have the same or similar effects (Kamiya, et al., 2013).

3. Age-Related Macular Degeneration

Age-related macular degeneration is the most common cause of irreversible central vision loss in elderly people. As the name suggests, it is caused by degeneration of the **macula**.

Dry Age-Related Macular Degeneration

Dry AMD occurs slowly and painlessly over a period of years and accounts for over 90% of AMD cases. In dry AMD, vision loss is gradual and usually occurs in both eyes. There is a gradual breakdown of the light-sensitive cells in the macula, and of the supportive tissue found under the macula.

The exact reason *why* dry AMD occurs is still unknown, but there are some solid theories. The layer under the retina, the retina epithelium (or 'skin'), may be affected by deposits of proteins, **oxidative stress**, and other age-related changes, such as a natural

59

thinning of the macula.

Waste product from the retina naturally accumulates in the epithelium (or 'skin') of the retina. This waste product is a yellow, fatty protein called **drusen**. Drusen can be either *hard* (found in tight, small patches throughout the eye), or *soft*. It is this soft stuff that has been identified as a risk factor for AMD. As the waste product accumulates, it causes changes to the pigment, rods, and cones (photoreceptors) of the retina.

During early stages, the patches of soft drusen are only about the thickness of a human hair and there is usually no vision loss. This can be detected during an eye exam by an ophthalmologist. Intermediate AMD is diagnosed when there are large drusen patches and changes to the pigment – by this stage, many people experience some vision loss, but others may not have noticed anything different in their vision at all.

In late AMD, drusen has accumulated in such large and heavy patches that it damages the macula. This causes a significant loss of central vision. There will be blurring when directly looking at something.

Signs & Symptoms of Dry AMD:
- Difficulty seeing (particularly reading) at night or in changing light conditions
- Fluctuating vision – some days are better than others!
- Difficulty reading or making out facial features
- Vision becomes 'wavy' – when looking at a grid of straight lines, some lines appear to bend, or parts of the grid may appear blank. This can be a useful way to monitor vision in AMD (see Appendix 1: Amsler Grid).

Dry AMD is also known as 'geographic atrophy' or 'non-exudative AMD'.

Wet Age-Related Macular Degeneration
Wet AMD is much less common than dry AMD. It is usually, but not always, preceded by the dry form. When the eye is damaged

by dry AMD, it sends a signal to the body that the retina needs more blood – probably in an effort to supply nutrients and oxygen to repair the damage. The vascular system responds to the signal and begins to build new blood vessels to the retina. This process is called 'neovascularisation' (*neo* = new; *vascularisation* = formation of blood vessels). Unfortunately, the new blood vessels are often fragile, abnormal, and 'leaky'. Blood, proteins, and fluids spill out of the vessels and accumulate beneath the macula, causing swelling, increased pressure, and large patches of scar tissue. This quickly causes rapid and severe damage and leads to sudden and irreversible vision loss.

Fluid can also leak from other areas of the eye and collect between areas in the retina. This build-up of fluid can cause a bump in the macula, leading to vision loss.

Signs & Symptoms of Wet AMD:
- Sudden vision changes in one eye
- Vision rapidly getting worse
- General haziness over vision
- Straight lines appear to bend or warp
- Difficulty seeing colours or fine details

It is possible to have both dry and wet AMD at the same time, and either condition can appear first.

Risk Factors for AMD:
- Age. Anyone over the age of 50 is at risk of age-related macular degeneration
- Genetics and family history
- Smoking
- High blood pressure
- Cardiovascular disease
- Obesity
- High levels of UV ray exposure from sunlight
- Dietary factors – low intake of omega-3 essential fatty acids and dark leafy green vegetables

AMD & the Age-Related Eye Disease Study

While there is no way to reverse the damage caused by dry AMD, conventional treatment includes nutritional supplementation to prevent its progression. In 2001, the Age-Related Eye Disease Study (AREDS) reported that a combination of nutrients called the 'AREDS formulation' can reduce the risk of developing advanced forms of AMD. The same researchers followed up their work with another study in 2006. Called AREDS2, this further refined the formulation and confirmed that nutritional medicine has a major role in preventing advanced AMD. Patients with drusen patches, pigment changes, or signs of eye changes can reduce their risk of developing advanced AMD by 25% by taking a combination of **zinc**, **copper**, **vitamin E**, **vitamin C**, **lutein**, and **zeaxanthin**.

The initial AREDS formulation:
- Beta-carotene 15mg
- Zinc 80mg
- Copper 2mg
- Vitamin C 500mg
- Vitamin E 400IU

The refined and improved AREDS2 formulation:
- Lutein 10mg
- Zeaxanthin 2mg
- Zinc 25mg or 80mg (25mg preferred as it's just as effective as 80mg and safer, with side effects and toxicity less likely)
- Copper 2mg
- Vitamin C 500mg
- Vitamin E 400IU

The AREDS and AREDS2 are considered landmark studies and their recommendations are the gold standard for nutrition in AMD. Despite the scope of these studies and the anecdotal positive effects that nutritional supplements can have on age-related macular degeneration, many people are non-compliant in taking supplements, even if a doctor or ophthalmologist recommends that they do so. Moreover, a 2016 study gave a questionnaire to 193 patients with age-related eye disease and found that 56% of the patients had not received any advice from their ophthalmologist about supplements and didn't even know taking them was an option! (Parodi, et al., 2016).

Lutein, Zeaxanthin & Meso-Zeaxanthin

These three antioxidants are found together in high concentrations in the **macular pigment** where they absorb blue light and protect the macula against oxidative damage. They are sometimes referred to as the 'macular carotenoids'. Research has shown that having a greater concentration of these nutrients in the macular pigment can slow down the accumulation of drusen and reduce the risk of AMD (Schleicher, et al., 2013). A large study involving five ophthalmology centres in the US showed that a higher dietary intake of lutein and zeaxanthin is associated with reduced AMD risk (Seddon, et al., 1994).

Many studies of nutritional supplements only include lutein and zeaxanthin, but recent research has found that these work best when combined with meso-zeaxanthin. A 2012 study found that supplementing with all three macular carotenoids was more effective at strengthening the macular pigment when compared to supplementing with just lutein and zeaxanthin (Loughman, et al., 2012). Unfortunately, neither the AREDS nor the AREDS2 investigated meso-zeaxanthin as it was discovered later than lutein and zeaxanthin. Based on what we know about meso-zeaxanthin, it is likely that the addition of meso-zeaxanthin 10mg to the AREDS2 formulation would be highly beneficial in further reducing the risk of advanced AMD.

Zinc

The first AREDS, in 2001, found that participants who took zinc supplements either alone or in combination with other nutrients were significantly less likely to develop advanced age-related macular degeneration (Age-Related Eye Disease Study Research

Group, 2001). The Blue Mountains Eye Study, a population-based study, confirmed that zinc can help to prevent disease progression in AMD patients (Tan, et al., 2008). Furthering this line of research, the 2011 Rotterdam Study found that zinc can regulate the genes associated with AMD and recommended that younger people at risk of AMD start taking zinc as soon as possible (Ho, et al., 2011). A 2014 study found that zinc influences the immune system to prevent changes to **lens proteins** and that 50mg of zinc sulphate per day can protect against the changes that could lead to AMD (Smailhodzic, et al., 2014).

However, a large review in 2013 concluded that zinc taken on its own may not be enough to prevent the onset or progression of age-related macular degeneration. The researchers acknowledged that the nutrients used in the AREDS studies, including zinc, may only work when they are taken together (Vishwanathan, et al., 2013). AREDS2 also found that a dose of 25mg of zinc per day was as effective as the larger 80mg dose used in the original AREDS (Aronow & Chew, 2015).

Note that the AREDS formulations include both copper and zinc – these minerals interact with each other and adequate levels of both are required for eye health. Too much zinc can cause a copper deficiency – the AREDS formula contains copper in order to prevent that from happening.

Vitamin C

The underlying mechanisms behind AMD include increased drusen production and immune cell activation. The damage that drusen patches cause to the macula is driven by free radicals, lipid peroxidation, and **oxidative stress**. Antioxidant nutritional and herbal medicines can intervene at many check-points of these cascades and stop their progression.

Vitamin C is the body's most abundant antioxidant and has a major role in preventing the progression of AMD. By quenching single oxygen free radicals, vitamin C can protect against the oxidative damage associated with AMD. The research agrees –

AMD is often seen in people who have a low dietary intake of vitamin C, and boosting intake of vitamin C can reduce the risk of developing AMD, particularly when taken in combination with **zinc** (Aoki, et al., 2016). Conventional treatment suggests that daily supplementation of 500mg is adequate to help prevent intermediate AMD or its progression to advanced AMD. Higher levels may be required in people with an increased need (e.g. the elderly, people with chronic illnesses, or athletes).

Antioxidants work in synergy with one another and appear together throughout nature. Studies show that a combination of multiple antioxidants is far more effective than just taking one alone. Many antioxidants are able to regenerate or 'recycle' each other. Some of these work in the aqueous or 'watery' environments of the body while others work in the lipid or 'fatty' areas, such as within cell membranes. A combination of vitamin C with other antioxidants could help to fight against the onset or progression of AMD.

Vitamin E
Vitamin E is routinely used as part of a multi-vitamin programme to prevent the progression of age-related macular degeneration, but there is very little experimental evidence that supports its use as an isolated supplement.

A large-scale, ten-year randomised trial of female participants showed that taking 600IU of supplemental vitamin E had neither a harmful nor beneficial effect on the risk of age-related macular degeneration (Christen, et al., 2010). It just didn't affect it at all!

An earlier trial found similar results in participants who took 500IU (containing 335 mg d-α tocopherol) per day for four years (Taylor, et al., 2002).

These unimpressive results may be due to the fact that vitamin E works more effectively when paired with other antioxidants.

B-Group Vitamins
The link between B vitamins and eye health is a little complex and centres around their role in cardiovascular health. We know

that people with cardiovascular disease are more likely to develop AMD – this is probably due to shared risk factors, like family history, as well as certain biochemical pathways that are activated throughout the body in both diseases. For example, high levels of **homocysteine** are linked to both cardiovascular disease *and* AMD.

Homocysteine is an amino acid. It is produced in the body through the metabolism of methionine, another amino acid. While homocysteine is a natural by-product of metabolism, it promotes inflammation and free radical damage. High levels have been linked directly to diseases that involve **oxidative stress** – particularly those that affect the circulatory system and **microcirculation**, such as atherosclerosis (where arteries become clogged with fatty substances) and age-related macular degeneration!

As we know, the retina is particularly sensitive to **oxidative stress** from UV radiation, by-products of normal cellular function, and the build-up of drusen deposits. While the body can generally maintain an even ratio of oxidative stress versus antioxidant activity, high levels of homocysteine may throw things out of balance. Homocysteine is an oxidative agent that can make any stress-induced injury worse. This means that it can exacerbate any damage already present in the tissues and blood vessels. This is common to both atherosclerosis and age-related macular degeneration. While atherosclerosis affects larger blood vessels and the heart, the end result is the same – cellular injury, tissue damage and, eventually, organ dysfunction.

Controlling homocysteine levels can reduce the risk of both cardiovascular disease and AMD. This is where B-group vitamins come in. The only way to reduce homocysteine levels is to convert it back into methionine, or to another amino acid called cysteine. Vitamin B12, folate, and vitamin B6 are essential for those pathways to work.

Research backs up the use of these three key B-group vitamins for the prevention of AMD. One seven-year study on the effects of taking B-group vitamins on AMD, for example, recruited over 5,000 women with cardiovascular risk factors. In particular, the researchers investigated the B-group vitamins that are essential for the metabolism of **homocysteine**. The study found that taking a combination of supplemental folic acid – a form of folate – (2.5mg), vitamin B6 (50mg), and vitamin B12 (1mg) per day was very effective at reducing homocysteine levels and, most importantly, can prevent the onset and development of AMD (Christen, et al., 2009).

NOTE: B-group vitamins work synergistically. It is important to take a general B-group supplement while taking higher doses of vitamin B12, folate, and vitamin B6.

Vitamin D

Vitamin D deficiency is related to an increased risk of age-related macular degeneration. There are a huge number of vitamin D receptors and associated enzymes found in the retina, suggesting that this prohormone plays an essential role in the healthy function of the retina and macula.

Vitamin D has been shown to control drusen levels, balance the immune system, influence the rate of cell replication and cell health, and inhibit oxidative stress and inflammation (Layana, et al., 2017). All of this helps to prevent the damage that causes both wet and dry AMD. A 2015 study showed that low vitamin D levels are associated with an increased risk of AMD, while high vitamin D levels are associated with decreased prevalence (Reins & McDermott, 2015).

Vitamin D has an especially key role in preventing wet AMD. It stops the formation of weak, chaotic blood vessels that leak fluids and proteins beneath the macula. By boosting vitamin D levels, dry AMD patients can strengthen their blood vessels and may prevent the onset of wet AMD.

There is one major issue with vitamin D, however – the sun. While UV rays are required for the body to produce vitamin D, exposure to UV rays from the sun actually increases the risk of developing

AMD. The answer here is to get *moderate* sun exposure and take vitamin D supplementation as necessary. Luckily, it is very easy and quite accurate to test vitamin D levels through a simple blood test. This can indicate whether supplementation is appropriate and safe. Speak to your doctor or nutritionist for more information and personalised advice.

Omega-3 Fatty Acids

The omega-3 fatty acids EPA and DHA help to moderate inflammatory processes – these inflammatory processes have been implicated in AMD. Many studies of various populations have shown that a high intake of EPA and DHA omega-3s, found in oily fish, is associated with a reduced risk of AMD (Seddon, et al., 2006; SanGiovanni, et al., 2007).

These findings were backed up by the landmark AREDS, which found that people with a high consumption of omega-3 were around 30% less likely to develop advanced AMD compared to those with a low intake (SanGiovanni, et al., 2009). Surprisingly, the AREDS2 study did not find omega-3 *supplementation* to further reduce the risk of developing advanced AMD when added to the original AREDS formula (Age-Related Eye Disease Study 2 (AREDS2) Research Group, 2013). Further reviews suggest that AREDS2 was not designed to adequately investigate the beneficial effects of omega-3 in AMD (Souied, et al., 2016). Given that many studies have shown the favourable link between a high intake of omega-3 and lower risk of AMD, taking EPA and DHA omega-3 supplements is likely to be beneficial, especially if you have a low consumption of oily fish.

Lycopene

Unlike the other carotenoids, lycopene is not concentrated in the macular pigment. However, it still plays a huge role in preventing the onset and progression of age-related macular degeneration. Population studies have shown that a high intake of lycopene can protect against AMD (Wu, et al., 2015). Its antioxidant activity can put a stop to a long list of inflammatory pathways that damage the retina and it may absorb light waves that would otherwise cause **oxidative stress** around the macula. Lycopene also strengthens blood vessels, which can prevent the progression of dry AMD into wet AMD by stopping fluid flowing into the eye (Mordente, et al., 2011).

Its major role in AMD may be as a back-up for lutein and zeaxanthin. A 2005 study found that AMD patients had much lower levels of lycopene, but that their levels of lutein and zeaxanthin were normal (Cardinault, et al., 2005). This can occur when lycopene donates electrons and essentially sacrifices itself to sustain the antioxidant powers of the other carotenoids. Again, this demonstrates that the power of taking multiple carotenoids together far outweighs the effects of taking just one or two in isolation.

Less Sodium

Hypertension (high blood pressure) is a risk factor for AMD, so anything that reduces blood pressure can reduce the risk of AMD, right? Not quite...

Common blood pressure medications do *not* reduce the risk of AMD and can even increase it, suggesting that lifestyle modifications are more relevant and useful (Etminan, et al., 2008; Klein, et al., 2014; McCarty, et al., 2001). The most commonly recommended lifestyle intervention that has real effects on both blood pressure *and* AMD risk is reducing sodium intake.

A high intake of dietary salt and low intake of water increases the pull of water and minerals *out* of the cells and into the blood. The heart has to 'push' harder to pump this larger volume of blood, which leads to hypertension. It's possible that this 'pull' can also add to the risk of wet AMD, where the sodium may encourage leakage from the blood vessels behind the macula.

Keeping an eye on salt in your diet is an easy way to control sodium intake. A 2016 study found that a daily salt intake of 5-8g daily is the sweet spot to aim for. This amount may effectively reduce hypertension *and* the risk of AMD. Don't go overboard though – less than 5g of salt per day can actually *increase* the risk. Boosting the amount of water you drink throughout the day can further balance the fluid throughout the body and within the eye (Bringmann, et al., 2016).

Carbohydrates

High blood sugar or **hyperglycaemia** can lead to the **glycation** of macular proteins. The Nurses' Health Study examined food diaries kept over a ten-year period by participants who were going to be assessed for age-related macular degeneration. In 2006, researchers analysed the data and found a strong connection between the glycaemic index of foods in the diet and the risk of developing AMD. Diets with a lot of high glycaemic index (GI) foods caused an increased risk of AMD. The researchers didn't find any connection between the total amount of carbohydrates consumed, *just* the quality of the carbohydrates (Chiu, et al., 2006). High GI foods are carbohydrate-rich foods that spike the blood sugar levels because they contain little fibre or fat to slow down the absorption of glucose into the circulation.

An analysis of the AREDS studies also concluded that people at risk of developing AMD or advanced AMD may benefit from eating smaller amounts of carbohydrates that are refined or have a high GI (Chiu, et al., 2007).

4. Dry Eye Syndrome

Technically called 'keratoconjunctivitis sicca', dry eye syndrome can be a symptom of many other health conditions, but can also occur without any other identifiable underlying causes. While dry eye syndrome isn't a significant threat to vision, it is the most common complaint that people visit the ophthalmologist about and it affects over 68% of people over the age of 60.

There are two main types of keratoconjunctivitis sicca – it can be caused by either an inadequate *quality* or an inadequate *quantity* of tears to lubricate the eye. Your optometrist or ophthalmologist will be able to examine your eyes and determine which form of dry eye syndrome you have.

Inadequate Tear Volume

In 'aqueous tear-deficient keratoconjunctivitis', the **lacrimal gland** doesn't produce enough tear fluid. Think of it as a kind of tear deficiency. It is the watery, or aqueous, part of tears that the lacrimal gland struggles to produce, leaving the surface of the eye insufficiently hydrated. As a result, the surface of the eye feels gritty and becomes susceptible to infection.

This form of dry eye syndrome can occur in isolation, but it is also a common symptom of certain conditions, such as viral infections, hepatitis C, HIV, lymphoma, and autoimmune conditions including Sjögren syndrome, rheumatoid arthritis, and lupus. Less commonly, it may be caused by conditions that involve scarring of the lacrimal gland, such as trachoma (a bacterial eye infection that can lead to blindness).

As well as the common symptoms of dry eyes (discussed below), the conjunctiva may appear dry and lustreless in this type of dry eye syndrome.

Evaporative Dry Eyes

In 'accelerated evaporation keratoconjunctivitis', or evaporative dry eyes, the lacrimal gland produces plenty of the watery component of tear fluid but the **meibomian glands** fail to supply adequate amounts of the lipids (the 'oily' component of tears). Normally, the oil keeps the tears stable and slows down their evaporation. Without this oil, the tears become too 'watery' and thin; this water is easily evaporated, leaving the surface of the eye insufficiently hydrated.

In this form, there is an abundance of tear fluid and possibly foam at the eyelid margin.

Inflammation is an underlying mechanism behind problems with the lacrimal and meibomian glands in either type of dry eye syndrome.

Symptoms of Dry Eyes:
- An itching or burning sensation in the eyes
- A feeling of having grit or a foreign body in the eye, or a

pulling sensation when moving the eye
- Worse in sunlight
- Sharp stabbing eye pain
- Eyestrain
- Fatigue
- Headaches
- Blurred vision
- Flood of tears after irritation

Generally speaking, symptoms fluctuate across the course of a day and are intermittent. They are often worse after prolonged visual effort, such as watching television, reading, driving, working on the computer, or using a smart-phone. General dehydration and environmental factors can also exacerbate the symptoms, particularly dryness, dust, wind, and smoky air.

Vitamin D

Vitamin D has a direct effect on the quality of tear production. A 2015 study found that a low level of vitamin D in the blood is linked to an increased risk of developing dry eye syndrome, while high levels may protect against its onset and progression (Reins & McDermott, 2015).

In 2016, a study examined the use of vitamin D injections as a treatment for cases of dry eye syndrome that weren't responding to conventional treatment options. The researchers recruited 105 patients who had tried medications and eye drops but still suffered from dry eye symptoms. They found that supplemental vitamin D injections increased the secretion and stability of the tears and reduced inflammation on the surface of the eye and along the eyelid margin. Most importantly, it improved all of the symptoms of dry eye syndrome (Bae, et al., 2016).

The following year, a smaller study found that oral vitamin D supplements hold just as much promise. After two months of supplementation with 1,000IU of vitamin D per day, participants with dry eye syndrome experienced a significant improvement in their symptoms and tear quality (Yang, et al., 2017).

Omega-3 Fatty Acids

Omega-3 essential fatty acids (EFAs) are required for the health and flexibility of all cellular membranes in the body. Two main omega-3s, EPA and DHA, keep inflammation in balance throughout the eye.

Researchers have found that higher dosages of EPA and DHA have better outcomes. One study compared the use of 325mg of EPA and 175mg of DHA to the use of a placebo, taken twice daily for three months. All participants in the omega-3 group experienced a significant improvement in their symptoms compared to the placebo group, particularly in respect of itching, burning, gritty sensation, and blurry vision (Bhargava, et al., 2013).

The source of omega-3s might be especially important. While fish oil has been considered the pinnacle of omega-3 supplementation for the last two decades, recent studies have shown that it is not always totally effective. A 2018 study trialled a fish oil supplement for the treatment of dry eye syndrome over 12 months and found that its effects were no better than a placebo (The Dry Eye Assessment and Management Study Research Group, 2018).

Conflicting study results over the last five years don't necessarily mean that omega-3 has no place in treating dry eye syndrome, however. Rather, it may highlight the issues with fish oil supplementation. While manufacturers attempt quality control, it is impossible to truly know the quality of omega-3s within each capsule; every fish harvested has a different level and quality of EPA and DHA that can be pressed into supplement form; many supplements remain in warehouses and on shop shelves for months before purchase; and fish oil becomes rancid relatively quickly once the bottle is open. So, there's no way to guarantee the quality of the omega-3 found in fish oil supplements. However, adding an antioxidant, such as vitamin E, can help prevent rancidity (Albert, et al., 2013).

Dietary intake of omega-3 is a good alternative and can quickly boost EPA and DHA levels. Fresh fatty fish provide pre-made EPA and DHA, while plant-based sources like walnuts, chia seeds, and hemp seeds require some additional metabolisation.

But that's only one piece of the puzzle. Ultimately the role of omega-3 is to balance out the pro-inflammatory pathways of omega-6 EFAs. Shifting the ratio of omega-3 to omega-6 in the diet can be as easy as eating more walnuts while cutting out foods that are rich in omega-6s – red meat, chicken, pork, ham, bacon, dairy, and eggs.

Omega-7 Fatty Acids

Research is still in its early stages, but animal studies have found that omega-7 fatty acids could help to cure dry eye syndrome. Oil from sea buckthorn pulp that is rich in omega-7 has been shown to improve the quantity *and* quality of tears by boosting the oil content of the fluids and nourishing the lacrimal glands. It has potent anti-inflammatory actions that can soothe the eyes, speed up recovery, and may even prevent acute bouts of dry eyes from turning into a chronic dry eye syndrome (Nakamura, S., et al., 2017).

Carbohydrates

A study in 2006 found that over 50% of people who had diabetes or were borderline diabetic reported that they suffered from chronic dry eye symptoms (Hom & De Land, 2006). **Hypergly-caemia** (high levels of glucose molecules in the blood) can cause damage to the lacrimal glands and dysfunction of the tear film. It also promotes inflammation, **oxidative stress**, and changes to the balance of **electrolytes** in the tear fluid. With a higher concentration of electrolytes in the fluid on the surface of the eye, water is quickly evaporated. This causes an osmolarity issue where the electrolyte concentration pulls water from the cells of the eye's surface, dehydrating those cells and causing damage to the tissues of the cornea (Zhang, et al., 2016).

Avoiding refined carbohydrates in the diet can help to control blood glucose levels and prevent hyperglycaemia. Whole grains and fibre-rich carbohydrate foods also tend to be packed full of other nutrients, such as B vitamins and magnesium, that are required to prevent other eye conditions.

Turmeric

Inflammation has been implicated as an underlying factor in dry eye syndrome. Chemical messengers that promote inflammation have been detected on the cornea of dry eye patients. Curcumin – a powerful anti-inflammatory component of turmeric – has been shown to inhibit the expression of these chemical messengers in animal studies (Chung, et al., 2012).

Curcumin has also been shown to protect the **electrolyte balance** and osmolarity of tear fluid. By maintaining the water balance in the tear fluid, curcumin can prevent the rapid removal of tears seen in evaporative dry eye syndrome. While research is still in its early stages, curcumin appears to promote healthy levels of oils in the tear film and helps to stop the liquid from drying out too quickly into the air (Chen, et al., 2010).

5. Cataracts

Cataracts are caused by changes to the proteins on the lens of the eye. These changes lead to an area of opacity in the otherwise transparent lens. People with cataracts may experience a gradual, painless blurring of the vision and other subtle symptoms. Most cases of cataracts are age-related and 30% of people in the UK over the age of 65 have cataracts – but they can occur at any age (Royal College of Ophthalmologists, 2010).

Lens changes are caused by damage to proteins and lipids (fats). These changes create an opacity that blurs the vision, causes irregular refractions of light and, eventually, creates blind spots. This damage can be caused by:

- UV rays that directly damage the lens proteins and generate free radicals
- **Oxidative stress** where there is an unequal balance of free radical activity to antioxidant supply
- **Glycation**, which occurs when sugars from carbohydrates damage lipids and proteins. Crystallins are pro-

teins that normally maintain the transparency of the lens but become opaque when they are damaged via glycation. Glycation is increased in **hyperglycaemia** and diabetics are at high risk of developing cataracts

- **Electrolyte imbalances**
- The ageing process, which naturally increases oxidative stress and protein changes (Khazaeni, 2017; Weikel, et al., 2014)

Signs & Symptoms of Cataracts:
Early

- Glare from oncoming light sources (such as headlights at night), or from brightly lit rooms or harsh sunlight. This is characterised as 'halos' and 'starbursts' appearing around the light sources. However, no pain is felt from the light
- Requiring more light to see well or to read accurately
- Difficulty distinguishing between blue and black colours

Late

- Painless blurring of total vision
- Eye strain and headache
- Development of short-sightedness, and possible improvement of close-range vision

Rare Complications

In very rare cases, the cataract can swell and push against the iris, resulting in pain and **closed-angle glaucoma**.

Risk Factors for Cataracts:

- Ageing
- Smoking
- Excessive alcohol use
- Long-term use of corticosteroids
- Inadequate nutrition
- Chronic exposure to ultraviolet light (e.g. long sun

exposure from working outdoors or driving every day)
- Exposure to x-rays
- Heat from infrared exposure
- Diabetes

Note that many cataract risk factors are modifiable lifestyle behaviours and addressing these risk factors can slow down the progression of existing cataracts. Many of the following underlying mechanisms involved in cataract formation can be addressed through nutritional interventions:

- **Free radical activity and oxidative stress** that contributes to changes to the lens fats and proteins. The eyes are exposed to lots of free radicals and oxidative stress from UV rays
- **Low levels of protective antioxidants**, including glutathione enzymes and nutrients like vitamin C and carotenoids. When there is a low amount of these antioxidants, the proteins and the membranes of the lens suffer from **oxidative damage**, leading to a change in the shape and structure of the lens
- **Osmotic imbalances & electrolyte disturbances.** Any issues with the fluid and mineral balance in the eye can impair the function of the membrane pump of eye cells. This causes a blockage to the in-flow of molecules, including antioxidants, that would otherwise be protecting the lens nucleus. Sodium, potassium, magnesium, and calcium are found in large concentrations in the lens – specifically with a ratio of low sodium to high potassium. Increases in sodium and calcium concentrations are seen in advanced cataracts and may cause changes to lens proteins (Chandorkar, et al., 1980; Mirsamandi, et al., 2004)
- **Hyperglycaemia** directly increases **oxidative stress** and **aldose reductase** (an enzyme that that converts glucose into **sorbitol**). Sorbitol further disrupts the **electrolyte balance** and increases the rate of **glycation,** leading to

further damage to the lens

Lutein, Zeaxanthin & Meso-Zeaxanthin

Lutein, zeaxanthin, and meso-zeaxanthin may be known as the macular carotenoids, but they are also present in large amounts in the lens. Here, they protect the proteins and fats against oxidation.

Lutein is well-researched for its role in preventing cataract onset and progression. It can even *improve* vision in people with established cataracts. A small two-year, double-blind placebo-controlled pilot study of 17 patients showed that, compared to vitamin E supplements or a placebo, taking 15mg of supplemental lutein three times a week resulted in improved vision in patients with cataracts (Olmedilla, et al., 2003).

Unfortunately, studies with larger numbers of participants and better study design suggest that the science may be a little more complicated. The Age-Related Eye Disease Study 2 (AREDS2) is a pinnacle research project that extended over five years. It continued from previous work conducted in the first AREDS, which found that nutritional intervention has a major role in treating many age-related eye diseases – including cataracts. However, AREDS2 showed that carotenoids may only help if the patient's baseline intake is already low. The five-year study of 3,159 elderly men and women found that taking 10mg of supplemental lutein along with 2mg of zeaxanthin each day did NOT significantly improve vision or have any marked effects on cataracts. The study did, however, find that the subgroup who had low baseline levels of these carotenoids from their diets experienced great improvements. They were the only group that had a lowered risk level of developing cataracts while they were taking the lutein and zeaxanthin supplements (Age-Related Eye Disease Study 2 (AREDS2) Research Group, et al., 2013).

More than anything, this demonstrates the need for adequate and consistent daily intake of carotenoids in the diet in order to prevent cataracts and to slow down their progression. These findings were also backed up by previous studies that showed that participants could lower their risk of advanced cataracts by eating a regular diet that included foods that are rich in lutein and zeaxanthin – particularly green leafy vegetables (Chasan-Taber, et al., 1999).

It's also possible that meso-zeaxanthin is the missing piece of the puzzle. Studies have shown that supplementing with an equal ratio of lutein, zeaxanthin, *and* meso-zeaxanthin is more effective in protecting the eye against oxidative damage than taking just one or two alone (Li, et al., 2010; Ma, et al., 2016).

Lycopene

Lycopene can protect against cataracts in a similar way to the other carotenoids. It can boost antioxidant activity in the lens and help the lens to remain translucent (Pollack, et al., 1985). Human trials are lacking, but animal studies show that lycopene clearly protects the eyes against cataracts (Gupta, et al., 2003).

People with **hyperglycaemia** and diabetes commonly have very low levels of lycopene. The high amounts of blood sugar in these populations can put high demand on **glycation** pathways so lycopene is used up trying to keep those pathways balanced. This bright red carotenoid has been shown to shut down glycation pathways by inhibiting the **aldose reductase** enzyme. In this way, lycopene can protect the lens against glycation protein changes and studies have shown that it helps the eyes to retain their translucency (Petyaev, 2016).

B-Group Vitamins

Each of the B-group vitamins has a role in protecting the eyes against cataracts. Not only do they supply the energy required for healthy cell function and turn-over but they have effects on the whole body that help to support the health of the eye. B vitamins are needed for healthy glucose metabolism, to prevent the accumulation of advanced **glycation** end products, and to boost glutathione levels.

Levels of B vitamins are typically low in older populations, who are at higher risk of developing cataracts.

A study of over 12,000 participants showed that higher niacin (vitamin B3) intake correlated with a lower risk of cataracts, as did a daily intake of at least 2 μg of riboflavin (vitamin B2). Supplementation of these two B vitamins reduced the risk of cataracts, particularly in populations with generally low or insufficient dietary intakes (Chiu & Taylor, 2007).

Vitamin B12, vitamin B6, and folate (vitamin B9) have a more complicated relationship with cataract prevention. As mentioned in the section on **age-related macular degeneration,** these B vitamins are essential for the metabolism of **homocysteine**, a key marker of cataract risk. Homocysteine has been shown to promote oxidative damage to the eye tissues and has been associated with juvenile **cataracts** (formation of cataracts in younger people). A 2008 study looked at the levels of homocysteine, vitamin B12, and folate in patients with cataracts. Sure enough, it found a low level of B12 and folate and a correspondingly high level of homocysteine in the patients who had the most advanced cataracts (Sen, et al., 2008). Taking supplemental doses of these B vitamins while adopting lifestyle changes can help to reduce homocysteine levels and the associated risk of developing cataracts.

It's important to remember that B vitamins work synergistically – for maximum effect, they must be taken in combination with one another, usually as a 'vitamin B complex' or 'vitamin B compound'.

Vitamin C

It is possible to boost the amount of vitamin C found in the eye tissues and aqueous humour by taking oral vitamin C supplements and/or increasing intake of vitamin C-rich foods in the diet. Green leafy vegetables are an important source of vitamin C, and these have been clearly associated with a decreased risk of cataracts and blindness in at-risk populations (Moïse, et al., 2012).

Vitamin C is abundant in the eye tissues and has a key role in maintaining healthy lens transparency. It is a potent antioxidant with direct free radical scavenger activity to protect the aqueous humour and lens against **oxidative stress** and **lens protein changes.** It also creates and regenerates glutathione antioxidant enzymes and regenerates other antioxidants, such as the **carotenoids**.

Vitamin C can protect the sodium-potassium pump to help regulate **electrolyte balance** throughout the eye. It also reduces the risk of **glycation** and **lens protein changes** by inhibiting a **glycation** enzyme, **aldose reductase**. Due to these direct actions in the lens, a high intake of vitamin C via the diet is strongly associated with lower odds of developing cataracts in population studies from around the world (Ravindran, et al., 2011; Valero, et al., 2002). However, supplementation isn't so promising. A large-scale random double-blinded placebo-controlled trial looked at the effects of daily vitamin C supplementation on healthy, older men without cataracts. Taking a dose of 500mg of vitamin C per day for eight years did not significantly reduce the risk of developing cataracts (Christen, et al., 2010).

Why would supplementation have *less* of a protective effect than vitamin C from food? People with high dietary intakes of vitamin C generally eat a diet that is rich in fresh fruits and vegetables – foods that also contain other key nutrients like **lutein** and **zeaxanthin** (García-Closas, et al., 2004). These antioxidants have been shown to work closely together with vitamin C to protect the whole body against oxidative stress and inflammation (Song, et al., 2015). It's probable that vitamin C needs to be taken together with other antioxidants, the way that they are found in nature, in order to protect the eyes against cataracts.

Vitamin E

Vitamin E is a fat-soluble antioxidant found in the fibres of the lens where it acts as a direct free radical scavenger.

In an eight-year study published in 2010, healthy men who

took 400IU of supplemental vitamin E each day experienced no protection against cataracts compared to a group who took a placebo (Christen, et al., 2010). There are a few issues with this study – the dose is quite low for vitamin E, the study used only one synthetic form of vitamin E, and there was no accounting for other lifestyle issues that increase the need for vitamin E (such as smoking and alcohol intake). A four-year randomised control trial from 2004, however, also found that, even at a slightly higher dose of 500IU per day, supplemental vitamin E had no protective effect against cataracts. In this study, the form of vitamin E was not discussed (McNeil, et al., 2004).

There is a bright side! A more recent meta-analysis from 2015 also agreed that vitamin E supplementation does not significantly protect against age-related cataracts, but dietary vitamin E intake *does* (Zhang, et al., 2015). This is possibly because the mixed tocopherols found in nature work in synergy.

Less Sodium

High levels of sodium in the diet can directly affect the levels of sodium found in the lens. A 2004 study found much higher levels of sodium and lower levels of potassium in patients with cataracts compared to those with healthy eyes (Mirsamadi, et al., 2004).

Electrolyte imbalances occur when the ratio of sodium to potassium is thrown out of balance and can lead to a dysfunction of the sodium-potassium pump on cellular membranes. This causes a blockage to the flow of antioxidants that could be protecting the lens, and an accumulation of waste products that can cause changes to lens proteins. Diets with excessively high levels of salt are a major risk factor for high blood pressure which, in turn, is a major risk factor for cataracts. High pressure in the blood vessels can cause **microcirculation issues**, increase pressure within the eye, and promote **oxidative stress** (Yu, et al., 2014).

Carbohydrates

You don't have to be diabetic to be at risk of cataracts from eating a high-carbohydrate diet. The quality and quantity of carbohydrate in the diet directly affects blood glucose levels. A high intake of refined carbohydrates, such as bread, sweets, cakes, chips, soft drinks, and lollies is associated with a risk of **hyperglycaemia** and may increase **glycation** processes in the lens. Healthy wholefood carbohydrate choices, such as vegetables, whole grains (e.g. brown rice), and legumes contain fibre that slows down the rate of sugar released into the blood, preventing **hyperglycaemia**.

However, it is essential to eat a balanced diet of healthy carbohydrates in moderation and balance them with fats and proteins. The *total* amount of carbohydrate in the diet has also been linked to cataract risk. A 2007 ten-year study showed that a diet with a high glycaemic load (i.e. high amounts of carbohydrates) was a risk factor for cataracts and a later study of 1,609 non-diabetic patients found a direct link between the level of carbohydrates – even 'healthy' ones – in the diet and the risk of developing cataracts! (Tan, et al., 2007; Chiu, et al., 2010).

Turmeric

The antioxidant properties of turmeric can combat **oxidative damage** in the lens that contributes to the development of cataracts. Specifically, studies show that a major active constituent within turmeric, curcumin, boosts the antioxidant enzymes, such as superoxide dismutase and glutathione, in the eye to prevent the formation of cataracts (Manikandan, et al., 2010).

Turmeric can also improve the function of nutrients that are linked to preventing cataract formation and progression. For example, turmeric has been shown to increase the concentration and activity of vitamin C levels in the lens (Murugan & Pari, 2006).

This bright orange root may also have a role in stopping cataract lens changes that are caused by advanced **glycation** end products and **blood glucose** issues. In two animal studies, curcumin extract was shown to prevent protein changes in the lens that lead to cataracts, particularly in animals with diabetes (Kumar, et al., 2005; Suryanarayana, et al., 2005).

Cataracts may be partially due to damage to the membranes of cells in the lens. This kind of damage creates a cascade of abnormal changes to the metabolism and composition of the lens and is one of the earliest signs of cataract formation. *In vitro* studies show that curcumin can promote the healthy apoptosis (programmed cell death) of human lens cells, clearing out damaged cells and allowing new, healthy lens cells to grow in their place (Hu, et al., 2012).

6. Glaucoma

Glaucoma is caused by progressive damage to the optic nerve and eventually results in blindness. Over 50% of people are unaware that they have glaucoma and it is the second-most common cause of blindness *worldwide*, not just within developing nations. Glaucoma is also the second leading cause of blindness within the UK, USA, and Australia.

Glaucoma can occur at any age, but the risk increases as the years progress and it is most common in people over the age of 60.

The optic nerve conveys visual information from the eye to the brain. Within the optic nerve are small cells called **retinal ganglion cells**, which also exist on the inner surface of the retina. These cells receive information from photoreceptors (light detectors), translate the light into images, and transmit it down their long **axons** (kind of like limbs), along the optic nerve and, finally, to the parts of the brain that process visual images.

The optic nerve and retinal ganglion cells are sensitive to changes in intraocular pressure. The eye is filled with aqueous humour, a fluid that is usually filtered out of the eye through a structure called the **trabecular meshwork** and drained back into circulation. Any issues affecting this process can lead to the two types of glaucoma – open-angle/wide-angle glaucoma and closed-angle glaucoma.

Open-Angle/Wide-Angle Glaucoma

In open-angle, or wide-angle, glaucoma, the flow of the aqueous humour is reduced or blocked at the trabecular meshwork. This meshwork is an area of spongy tissue located at the base of the cornea. When the trabecular meshwork becomes obstructed, it causes a backlog of aqueous humour and a chronic, painless build-up of pressure within the eye (also known as 'intraocular pressure'). This increased intraocular pressure damages the optic nerve by either directly compressing the axons of the retinal ganglion cells or by compressing the blood vessels that supply the optic nerve with oxygen and nutrients.

However, the relationship between intraocular pressure and glaucoma is complicated. Only 10% of people with high intraocular pressure (or 'ocular hypertension') will develop glaucoma. At the same time, over a third of people with glaucoma do *not* have ocular hypertension. There is also research and speculation about other factors that may contribute to the degradation of the optic nerve, such as immune system dysfunction, **oxidative stress** and free radical damage, and **microcirculation issues** causing reduced blood flow to the optic nerve.

Signs & Symptoms of Open-Angle Glaucoma:

- Often undetected until late stages
- Painless, progressive, and patchy loss of vision
- Hazy or blurred vision
- The appearance of rainbow-coloured circles around bright light sources
- Often affects the peripheral vision and general vision is preserved until the disease is advanced. This highlights the need for yearly eye examinations by an optometrist who can test the intraocular pressure in the eyes

Closed-Angle Glaucoma

Closed-angle, or tight-angle, glaucoma is also believed to be associated with an increase of intraocular pressure. In this case, the flow of aqueous humour is blocked by the iris *before* it reaches the trabecular meshwork. This is usually sudden and painful.

Signs & Symptoms of Closed-Angle Glaucoma:

- Eye pain
- Headaches
- Halos around light sources
- Dilated pupils in all levels of light
- Vision loss
- Red eyes
- Nausea
- Vomiting

These symptoms last for hours, or until the intraocular pressure is released.

Risk Factors for Both Types of Glaucoma:

- Family history, particularly siblings or parents
- African-American or Latino heritage
- Diabetes
- Cardiovascular disease
- Age – a six-fold increase of risk after the age of 60

Vitamin A & Carotenoids

Vitamin A is a lipid-soluble antioxidant that is essential for membrane integrity. It has a particular benefit for the eye tissues and may help to maintain the healthy growth and development of the trabecular meshwork. Vitamin A supplements are rarely given, except in confirmed cases of a deficiency. This is because high doses of vitamin A can accumulate in the body and cause toxicity. Instead, 'retinol equivalents', such as beta-carotene or other carotenoids are prescribed. These can be converted into active vitamin A (retinol) by the body, without the risk of toxicity.

Retinol, whether from dietary vitamin A or beta-carotene, acts as an antioxidant in fatty environments, such as the membranes and epithelium of the trabecular meshwork. It helps to fortify the integrity of the meshwork and can protect it against degradation by reducing **oxidative stress**.

A cross-sectional study of almost 3,000 patients investigated the role of dietary factors, including vitamin A supplementation, and the risk of developing open-angle glaucoma. The study concluded that taking vitamin A or retinol equivalent supplements did not provide any *reduction* to the risk. However, this conclusion was based on a survey that asked patients to self-report on any dietary supplements that they had taken in the previous 30 days but it did *not* take dietary intake into consideration (Wang, et al., 2013). In short, the collection of data was sketchy at best!

On the other hand, the Rotterdam Study was a longitudinal study of 3,502 participants over a period of almost ten years. This benchmark study suggested that vitamin A levels have a key role in preventing glaucoma. The data showed that a low dietary intake of retinol equivalents was associated with a significantly higher risk of developing open-angle glaucoma (Ramdas, et al., 2012).

CAUTION: In current and former smokers, beta-carotene supplementation can increase the risk of lung cancer. Recently, the substitution of beta-carotene with other carotenoids, namely lutein and zeaxanthin, has been shown to have a comparable effect to beta-carotene.

Lutein, zeaxanthin, and **meso-zeaxanthin** are powerful antioxidant carotenoids that are found throughout the eye tissues and inside the trabecular meshwork. They may help to control oxidative stress that contributes to meshwork blockages and optic nerve damage (Mares, 2017).

Vitamin C

Vitamin C can protect against glaucoma by maintaining healthy intraocular pressure. It does this by maintaining the collagen structure of the trabecular meshwork, ensuring there is adequate space within the meshwork for a strong outflow of the aqueous humour. As an antioxidant, it can also prevent the accumulation of debris in the trabecular meshwork by reducing free radicals and quenching oxidative stress.

The available data supports its use in preventing both open- and closed-angle glaucoma. A 2013 population-based study found that taking a vitamin C supplement (at both low and high doses) was found to be associated with decreased odds of glaucoma (Wang, et al., 2013). A meta-analysis in 2018 also found that, after accounting for variables between the 36 articles that were analysed, vitamin C has a significant protective effect against glaucoma (Ramdas, et al., 2018).

B-Group Vitamins

While other nutrients protect against glaucoma by maintaining healthy intraocular pressure, B-group vitamins work directly to support and protect the optic nerve itself.

Thiamine (vitamin B1) is essential for the metabolism of carbohydrates into cellular ATP (adenosine triphosphate – the main source of energy for most cellular processes) to fuel the transmission of electrical signals through the optic nerve. A deficiency of vitamin B1 has been shown to degrade retinal ganglion cells, whereas a metabolite (product of metabolism) of vitamin B1 has been shown to have protective effects on the cells and their axons that send signals to the brain (Kang, et al., 2010).

If a deficiency of this B vitamin can increase the *risk* of glaucoma, can taking a supplement of the nutrient prevent it, even if you already have 'healthy' thiamine levels? Maybe...

One study from 2012 showed that taking supplemental thiamine has been associated with a decreased incidence of glaucoma (Ramdas, et al., 2012). However, a thorough meta-analysis by the same authors in 2018 concluded that it has only a mild protective effect (Ramdas, et al., 2018).

NOTE: Alcohol rapidly depletes thiamine and alcoholism is a major cause of vitamin B1 deficiency. However, no studies have found that alcoholism is directly related to the risk of glaucoma.

Vitamin D

A retrospective cross-sectional study looked at the data from 123,331 patients who had been screened for glaucoma and vitamin D deficiency between 2012 and 2013. The researchers found that low levels of vitamin D in the blood were significantly associated with a higher risk of developing glaucoma, particularly in women (Kim, et al., 2016).

The mechanism behind this may involve vitamin D's role in protecting DNA and regulating healthy cell division. It may also play into theories that the immune system is involved in blocking up the trabecular meshwork. Vitamin D regulates all immune cells and their functions and low levels of this prohormone can cause these cells to malfunction and leave debris within structures like the meshwork. This may explain why vitamin D was also shown to reduce intraocular pressure.

Vitamin E

Vitamin E is a tricky nutrient. As described in the **vitamin E** section earlier, vitamin E comes in a range of different compounds (tocopherols and tocotrienols) which are found together in nature. Unfortunately, studies rarely use a range of vitamin E compounds when looking at the effects of vitamin E supplementation. This may be one reason why studies have such radically different outcomes.

One ten-year study, for example, showed that people with higher intakes of supplemental vitamin E have an *increased* risk of glaucoma (Ramdas, et al., 2012). Conversely, a smaller study of only 12 months duration showed that participants who took vitamin E supplements were significantly *less likely* to develop glaucoma than those who did not (Ramdas, et al. 2018). Does it come down to the different forms of vitamin E? Maybe...

The data is clearer when it comes to treating glaucoma, rather than simply preventing it. A 2014 study showed that vitamin E supplementation *does* have a beneficial effect on the function of the retina in open-angle glaucoma patients and caused a subsequent improvement in vision after 6-12 months of treatment (Parisi, et al., 2014).

Magnesium

Magnesium is a vasodilator. It relaxes blood vessels so that more blood can flow through the **microcirculation**. This improves circulation to tight spaces, such as the eyes, delivering more nutrients and oxygen to nourish the optic nerve and trabecular meshwork.

An early study from 1995 found that taking magnesium could improve vision in patients with glaucoma by reversing the constricting effects on blood vessels from cold temperatures, which allowed more blood to reach the capillaries of the eyes (Gasper, et al., 1995). However, this study used only ten participants and only observed improvement after a very short follow-up. The researchers did not check to see if magnesium supplementation had effects in the long-term, so the study does not reflect the real-world impact of magnesium on glaucoma progression.

Conversely, the decade-long Rotterdam Study showed that magnesium supplementation was associated with an *increased* risk of glaucoma (Ramdas, et al., 2012), as did two other studies on blood pressure and glaucoma. (Langman, et al., 2005; Müskens, et al., 2007).

Eating magnesium-rich foods is less likely to contribute to this increased risk. Magnesium is found in small amounts in many foods, such as green leafy vegetables, that are also rich in antioxidants and other nutrients that have been shown to prevent glaucoma.

Turmeric

The exact mechanisms underpinning glaucoma remain unclear. Elevated intraocular pressure is the most critical risk for glaucoma and is reported to cause damage to the optic nerve by damaging retinal ganglion cells.

Curcumin (a major active constituent of turmeric) is neuroprotective, which means that it protects all types of nerve cells – including the optic nerve – and it may be effective in the prevention and treatment of glaucoma.

There is very little research currently available on the effects of turmeric or curcumin on glaucoma. However, in an animal study, pre-treatment with curcumin was able to increase nerve cell health and protect against **oxidative damage** to the retinal ganglion cells when intraocular pressure was raised (Yue, et al., 2014).

Carbohydrates

Refined carbohydrates are quick to be digested and release glucose molecules into the bloodstream. Also known as a blood sugar 'spike', this can cause an acute state of **hyperglycaemia.** Chronic hyperglycaemia is seen in uncontrolled diabetes. Any state of high blood sugar can increase the rate of **glycation** to proteins and lipids throughout the eye.

A 2008 study found that glycation products (the residues of proteins and lipids) are found in high amounts in the trabecular meshwork of patients with glaucoma (Zubaty, et al., 2008). These proteins and lipids that have undergone glycation (or 'advanced glycation end products') may be a major cause of blockages in the trabecular network, causing a back-up of aqueous humour and increased intraocular pressure. They have also been found in the optic nerve and retina in glaucoma patients (Tezel, et al., 2007).

Refined carbohydrate foods, such as cakes, lollies, sweets, and soft drinks are likely to cause blood glucose spikes and may contribute to glycation processes. Healthy carbohydrate choices that also include fibre, protein, and fat will maintain a steady, moderate level of sugar in the blood. This may help to protect against damage to the optic nerve (Zarnowski, et al., 2012).

Less Sodium

Sodium, mostly found in the diet as salt, can contribute to damage to the optic nerve by increasing blood pressure throughout the body. Any added pressure in the blood vessels near the eyes will push more pressure into the intraocular chamber.

A large study of over 27,000 patients with glaucoma found that people with high blood pressure were far more likely to be diagnosed with glaucoma than people with normal blood pressure (Langman, et al., 2005). Sodium intake is a major driving factor behind high blood pressure and reducing salt intake can help to manage the risk of hypertension *and* glaucoma. While most people in the UK consume 8g of salt per day, the NHS recommends that adults consume no more than 6g of added salt per day – that's about one teaspoon (NHS, 2017).

Avoid Caffeine

A 2011 systematic review and meta-analysis of the available evidence concluded that caffeine increases intraocular pressure in people with glaucoma. However, it does not appear to have any effect on intraocular pressure in people who do *not* have glaucoma (Li, et al., 2011). Why? No one knows. It is advisable, however, that people with glaucoma stay away from coffee, tea, and cola!

7. Night Blindness (Nyctalopia)

Night blindness or 'nyctalopia' is defined as a failure for the eyes to adapt promptly from light to dark conditions. This is often caused by **keratomalacia**, an eye condition caused by vitamin A deficiency and discussed shortly. Vitamin A deficiency causes the reduced photosensitivity of a protein called 'rhodopsin' that is found in retina cells. This causes a night blindness that is not usually severe, and vision most often recovers when vitamin A levels are adequately restored from supplementation.

Night blindness can also be due to congenital and inherited retinal disorders, diabetes, or as a 'secondary condition' to cataracts and glaucoma.

Signs & Symptoms of Night Blindness (Nyctalopia):

- Difficulty seeing in the dark, whether at night time or in dim rooms

- The first noticeable symptom is often difficulty driving at night
- More difficulty seeing when moving from a brightly lit environment to an area of low light

Risk Factors for Night Blindness (Nyctalopia):
- Vitamin A deficiency due to poor diet
- Other eye diseases such as **cataracts** and **glaucoma**
- **Myopia** (short- or near-sightedness)
- Family history
- Diabetes

Treatment for night blindness requires a clear diagnosis of the underlying conditions that are causing nyctalopia symptoms. Addressing night blindness alone will not resolve the core disease and could hazardously mask the true cause that requires treatment. Always seek advice from a doctor or ophthalmologist.

Vitamin A
Vitamin A deficiency and the subsequent onset of **keratomalacia** is a leading cause of night blindness. This condition leads to the degeneration of the cornea. Check your diet to ensure you are getting an adequate intake of **vitamin A** and see the section on **keratomalacia** for more information.

Bilberry
Bilberry extract is used in traditional western herbal medicine to treat a host of eye conditions, including night blindness. It is rich in tannins, flavonoids, anthocyanosides, and other antioxidants that have a high affinity for the retina. Its mechanisms of action include protecting the eye against **oxidative damage**, improving **microcirculation** (particularly in people with diabetes who are at risk of **hyperglycaemia**), and reducing inflammation throughout the body.

While there is very little literature on bilberry's effects, one double-blinded placebo-controlled study looked at the effects of this unique herb on night vision. The trial was small, with only six participants in each group, but all of those who took a standardised bilberry extract adapted to darkness significantly faster than those who took a placebo (Zafra-Stone, et al., 2007).

It's important to note that this study was *very* small and has limited validity because of its study design. This is a common problem with bilberry studies. In fact, a review of 30 published trials of bilberry extracts on lowered light and night vision found that there were issues with almost all published papers on the topic – for example, only 12 of the 30 published studies were placebo-controlled. The researchers writing the review concluded that there was insufficient rigorous evidence to recommend the use of bilberry for improving night vision (Canter & Ernst, 2004). That being said, herbal traditionists swear by its efficacy and there have been no studies showing any harm from taking moderate doses of bilberry.

8. Keratomalacia

Keratomalacia is an eye disorder caused by a vitamin A deficiency. It affects the cornea and the conjunctiva.

Vitamin A is needed for the proper growth and division of healthy cells. In particular, it is required to maintain the specialised tissues of the cornea and conjunctiva called 'epithelia'. The conjunctiva is a thin mucous membrane that covers the front of the eyeball and the inside of the eyelid. When there are inadequate levels of vitamin A, the soft, moisturised cells of the conjunctiva epithelia are replaced with rough, keratinised **cells** and there is also a destruction of mucus-producing **goblet cells**.

The purpose of mucus in the eye is two-fold – to lubricate the surface for smooth movement, and to protect the eyes against infectious pathogens. Without a smooth, mucosal surface, the conjunctiva becomes thick, wrinkled, and cloudy. Meanwhile, the cornea (the clear layer that forms the front of the eyeball) becomes softer and susceptible to infections that can cause corneal ulceration. In extreme cases, the conjunctiva and cornea can become completely overrun by fibrotic scar tissue.

Additionally, the lacrimal glands and the conjunctiva become irritated, resulting in further drying of the eyes and redness in the 'whites' of the eyes. Foamy spots can appear on the conjunctiva.

Signs & Symptoms of Keratomalacia:

- Severe dryness of the cornea and conjunctiva (also known as 'xerophthalmia')
- **Nyctalopia** (night blindness or difficulty seeing well in dimly lit spaces)
- Cloudiness in the corneas
- Foamy spots on the conjunctiva. Called 'Bitot's spots', these look like a build-up of light grey, foamy patches

Risk Factors for Keratomalacia:

- Vitamin A deficiency
- General malnutrition
- Inadequate protein intake
- Alcohol use
- Measles
- Pneumonia
- Liver disease
- Chronic diarrhoea
- Malabsorption conditions, such as coeliac disease
- Inflammatory bowel diseases
- Cystic fibrosis

Vitamin A

The front-line therapy for keratomalacia is, fairly obviously, vitamin A supplementation to quickly boost and maintain the levels in the body. While vitamin A deficiency was once considered a 'rare' condition in the developed world, recent research suggests that it is actually more common than previously thought. In undeveloped nations, vitamin A deficiency goes hand-in-hand with general malnutrition and low protein intake but in developed nations, the deficiency is usually caused by alcoholism, liver disease, and inflammatory bowel diseases – there are adequate amounts of vitamin A in the diet *but* there are factors stopping its absorption into the body. Good news: strategic supplementation can boost the levels of vitamin A in the blood, even if these other factors remain the same. In extreme cases of malabsorption conditions, vitamin A can be given as an injection into a muscle where it is then absorbed into the blood.

Once vitamin A levels are restored, many symptoms of mild-to-moderate keratomalacia may be reversed (Privett & Mahajan, 2011). Some patients who have chronic malabsorption conditions (e.g. coeliac disease) may need to maintain vitamin A supplementation to ensure their requirements are met. Speak to a qualified nutritionist for personalised advice.

9. Blepharitis

Blepharitis is an inflammatory condition that affects the eyelid margin. It can be acute (quick to present and quick to resolve) or chronic, and its origins can be infectious or non-infectious.

Infectious Blepharitis

Infectious blepharitis is usually caused by a bacterial or viral infection in the margin of the eyelid, where the lid meets the eyelashes. The follicles of the eyelashes and the meibomian glands (at the base of each lash) are also usually infected. It's easy to distinguish between bacterial and viral blepharitis by the colour and thickness of discharge in the eye. Bacterial infections tend to cause crusting, while viral blepharitis causes prolific, clear discharge. Infection is usually by *Staphylococcal* bacteria, or a herpes simplex, or varicella-zoster virus.

Additionally, bacterial blepharitis can actually be caused by mites – the *Demodex* mite carries *Staphylococcal* bacteria on the surface of its own body and it can cause physical irritation to the lid margin. This is known as Demodex blepharitis and it is one of the most common, but frequently overlooked, causes of infectious blepharitis. It is particularly common in people who also have **acne rosacea** – a condition involving the congestion of oil-glands, including those on the eyelid margin, leading to a perfect oily environment for *Demodex* mites to thrive (Liu, et al., 2010).

Signs & Symptoms of Infectious Blepharitis:
- Itching
- Burning
- Feeling of a foreign body on the eye
- Crusting of the lid margin (in bacterial blepharitis)
- Prolific, clear discharge (in viral blepharitis)
- Eyelids can feel 'stuck together' when waking up after sleep
- Redness of the lid margin
- Blurry vision
- Dandruff of the eyelashes
- Inflammation and swelling of the lid margin
- Meibomian gland dysfunction (leading to **dry eye syndrome**)

Symptoms of infectious blepharitis are usually **acute** with a sudden onset. The acute condition responds quickly to treatment, but some cases can reoccur and develop into chronic blepharitis. Recurrent acute blepharitis is inconvenient and uncomfortable but does not usually result in any scarring of the cornea or vision loss.

Non-Infectious Blepharitis
Chronic blepharitis, also known as non-infectious or seborrhoeic blepharitis, is the most common form of blepharitis in adulthood. It occurs when the glands at the base of the eyelashes become clogged. These are the meibomian glands that produce an oily substance that forms part of healthy tear film (see: **Dry Eye Syndrome**). Inflammation of the meibomian glands causes an obstruction of the gland outlets, leading to a build-up of oil which then becomes oxidised and forms a thick, waxy secretion.

Signs & Symptoms of Non-Infectious Blepharitis:
- Greasy, easily removable scales on the margins of the eyelids

- Pressing the meibomian glands causes them to expel a thick, waxy, yellowish secretion
- Dry eye symptoms, such a feeling of grittiness on the eye, foreign body sensation, eye strain, visual blurring, fatigue, and headaches

Vitamin D

There are limited studies available on the role of vitamin D in non-infectious blepharitis. However, one case report on two teenagers with blepharitis found that, along with a serious vitamin A deficiency, vitamin D deficiency played a role in the pathogenesis of the disease (Duignan, et al., 2015). This is likely due to vitamin D's essential role in maintaining immune defences against pathogens like mites, bacteria, and viruses.

Omega-3 Essential Fatty Acids

Omega-3 essential fatty acids are involved in regulating inflammation throughout the body and, more locally, they influence the health and composition of the oily liquids secreted by the meibomian glands. A low ratio of omega-3 to omega-6 EFAs can result in inflammation in and around the glands and cause them to produce a thicker, waxier secretion that can easily block the glandular ducts and cause blepharitis.

A 2008 study found that taking 1,000mg of omega-3 three times a day improved tear production and stability, supported general meibomian gland health, and caused a reduction of chronic blepharitis symptoms (Macsai, 2008).

A later study in 2014 investigated the effects of a supplement formulation that contained 500mg of omega-3, taken three times per day in a randomised, double-blind placebo-controlled trial. This unique study looked at the effects of the nutrient supplement on the quality of life of people with chronic blepharitis – this included mental health and sense of well-being, along with physical signs of inflammation and blepharitis symptoms. After three months of treatment, the participants who were taking the formulation experienced improvement in tear film stability and subsequent relief of dry eye symptoms, decreased inflammation along the lid margin, and a significant relief of emotional distress and discomfort (Oleñik, et al., 2014).

Eyebright

The name says it all! Eyebright is a herb that is traditionally used as an eyewash for eye diseases that present with signs of infection and inflammation. Bathing the eyes with eyebright can literally *brighten* the eyes... Or, at least, relieve redness, crusting, and lash dandruff! This herb is rich in antimicrobial constituents, including thymol and linalool, making it an ideal therapy for infectious blepharitis. The antimicrobial activity of the volatile oils within eyebright have strong antibacterial effects on pathogens that commonly cause eye infections, including *Staphylococcal aureus*, that can be responsible for blepharitis (Novy, et al., 2015).

Goldenseal

Goldenseal is another herbal medicine that is traditionally used to treat blepharitis as well as **conjunctivitis**. However, no published research is available on its efficacy. It is rich in berberine, a strong antibacterial alkaloid which *could* have positive effects on controlling *Staphylococcal aureus* bacterial infection associated with blepharitis. However, do NOT expose the eyes to bright sunlight after using goldenseal eyewashes or eye drops. A 2007 trial showed that berberine from goldenseal is phototoxic to human lens cells – this means that caution must be used when applying goldenseal topically, as the combination of goldenseal and sunlight can destroy the cells of the lens (Chignell, et al., 2007).

Tea Tree (*Melaleuca*)

Tea tree oil is another traditional herbal remedy for infectious blepharitis. This, though, has more recent research around its safety and efficacy.

A 2018 study of 40 participants looked into the effectiveness of tea tree oil versus a placebo in cases of chronic blepharitis. The patients who received a patented tea tree oil product were to apply the oil twice daily for two months, while the placebo group performed self-massage, without any oil, after applying a warm compress to the eye. All participants who used the tea tree oil product quickly showed improvement in symptoms, as well as a better quality of tears and greater lens lubrication. They reported having 'fresh eyes upon awakening in the morning'. Meanwhile, the placebo group did not experience any of these improvements, even after two months of using warm compresses and massage (Maher, 2018).

The effects of tea tree oil are likely to be antimicrobial, antiviral, *and* anti-mite! An earlier and larger study of 335 participants found that the use of an eye scrub containing tea tree oil was strongly linked to the relief of discomfort and a reduction in *Demodex* infection, especially compared to a placebo scrub that did not contain tea tree oil (Koo, et al., 2012). Tea tree oil is incredibly potent. To avoid irritation and even damage to the eye, tea tree oil should be well-diluted before applying topically.

10. Conjunctivitis

Conjunctivitis is a condition of inflammation of the conjunctiva. It is characterised by red conjunctiva and a weeping or thick discharge from the eye (or both eyes), which can dry into a crust overnight and 'glue' the eyelids shut. Conjunctivitis is usually acute, with a sudden onset, and is often caused by a viral or bacterial infection of the conjunctiva. It can, however, also be due to an allergic reaction or physical irritation.

Viral Conjunctivitis

Viral conjunctivitis is highly contagious. It is usually caused by adenoviruses or enteroviruses but is occasionally found alongside viral infections that affect the whole body such as chickenpox, measles, rubella, and mumps. It is also seen with upper respiratory tract infections, such as influenza.

Signs & Symptoms of Viral Conjunctivitis:

- Red conjunctiva
- Watery discharge
- Irritation in the eye

- Slightly swollen eyelid
- Usually begins in one eye and spreads to the other
- Pain in sunlight
- A feeling of something in the eye
- Blurred vision
- The conjunctiva may look swollen and gelatinous
- Lymph nodes located in front of the ear may be raised

Bacterial Conjunctivitis

Most bacterial conjunctivitis is acute with a rapid onset and a quick recovery. Generally speaking, *Staphylococcal aureus, Streptococcus pneumoniae,* and *Haemophilus* bacteria are the most common causes. However, *Chlamydia* bacteria can cause chronic conjunctivitis, which can lead to blindness, and *Neisseria gonorrhoeae* can cause gonococcal conjunctivitis after sexual contact with a person who has a gonorrhoea infection of the genitals.

Signs & Symptoms of Bacterial Conjunctivitis:

- Begins in one eye and spreads to the other within a few days
- A thick discharge that is yellow or white
- The conjunctiva appears red, swollen, and gelatinous
- Severe swelling of the eyelid
- Blurred vision
- Symptoms typically develop within 12-48 hours of exposure

Rare complications include corneal ulceration, abscesses, and blindness. It is important to seek medical treatment as soon as possible to prevent these complications.

Allergic Conjunctivitis

Also known as atopic conjunctivitis, the allergic form of conjunctivitis typically flares-up seasonally or when exposed to particular airborne allergens. It is easy to tell if you have allergic conjunctivitis rather than viral or bacterial types – the allergic form involves extreme itchiness of the eyes.

Seasonal allergic conjunctivitis (hay fever conjunctivitis) is caused by airborne spores of mould, or pollen from grasses, trees, and weeds. Typically, people with seasonal allergic conjunctivitis suffer from symptoms during spring and summer and experience relief during autumn and winter, but this depends entirely on the life cycle of the plants and moulds that release the allergens.

Perennial allergic conjunctivitis (atopic conjunctivitis) is caused by non-seasonal, year-round allergens, such as dust mites, animal dander, and tobacco smoke. Symptoms can occur anytime throughout the year.

Vernal keratoconjunctivitis is a unique form of conjunctivitis that *may* be allergic. It generally appears each spring and summer and is more common amongst males from childhood to age 20 who have eczema, asthma, and seasonal allergies.

Signs & Symptoms of Allergic Conjunctivitis:

- Presents in both eyes from the start (does not spread from one to the other)
- Red conjunctiva
- Itchiness in the eyes
- Mild or moderate swelling of the eyelids
- Watery or stringy, clear discharge
- Often presents along with a stuffy, runny nose or eczema
- Conjunctiva can appear velvety
- Swelling of the eyelid and chronic eyelid rubbing can cause **blepharitis**

Vitamin D

With an essential role in immune cell regulation, the presence of vitamin D in the eye can protect against bacterial and viral causes of conjunctivitis and may also stabilise the immune system against allergic reactions. But how can you boost the level of vitamin D in the eye tissues and fluids?

It appears that oral supplementation will do the trick. In a study of 48 healthy volunteers, researchers found that the levels of vitamin D found in the blood were reflective of the levels found in the tear fluid. The study went even further and found that healthy tear fluid contains much *higher* amounts of vitamin D than is found in the blood. The researchers concluded that the eye fluids contain concentrated amounts of vitamin D to prevent diseases on the eye surface, such as infectious conjunctivitis (Sethu, et al., 2016).

The link extends to allergic forms of conjunctivitis, too. A case-control study of nearly 100 participants examined the connection between vitamin D levels and symptoms of seasonal allergic conjunctivitis. The researchers found that vitamin D levels were significantly lower in patients with seasonal allergic conjunctivitis than those without. This can indicate two possibilities (or a combination of them both):

- Vitamin D protects the eyes against allergic conjunctivitis, so people with low vitamin D levels have a higher risk of suffering from the condition
- Allergic conjunctivitis depletes the body of vitamin D

Whichever of these proves to be true, boosting vitamin D levels during bouts of conjunctivitis is highly recommended (Dadaci, et al., 2014).

Omega-7 Fatty Acids

Particular omega-7 fatty acids have been shown to have antibacterial activity in conjunctivitis. A 2017 study found that applying a topical blend of omega-7 fatty acids can destroy bacteria that cause gonorrhoeal conjunctivitis, even when the bacteria is resistant to conventional antibiotic medications. The study also showed that these fatty acids can protect the eyes against infection (Churchward, et al., 2017). The antioxidant effects of omega-7s may also help to repair any damage and speed up recovery from conjunctivitis.

Quercetin

Quercetin is an interesting antioxidant that has a unique action on the immune system. It is able to stabilise mast cells – the cells that release histamine, a chemical messenger that causes symptoms of allergic conjunctivitis. By stabilising the mast cells, the immune system is less likely to have a knee-jerk reaction to environmental allergens. Quercetin can also 'mop up' histamine to help relieve symptoms quickly.

A study in 2015 looked at the effects of a product containing quercetin, vitamin D3, and the extract of *Perilla frutescens* (a herb). The 23 participants all had allergic conjunctivitis and were given the product for one month. Approximately 70% of their symptoms were resolved within 30 days and there were no noteworthy side effects recorded. Whether this is due to the vitamin D, the quercetin, or the herbal medicine is unclear, but it could be a combination of all three (Ariano, 2015).

Eyebright

Eyebright is traditionally used as an eyewash for infectious conjunctivitis and **blepharitis.** It contains a high concentration of antimicrobial oils which have been shown to destroy bacteria that commonly cause eye infections, including *Enterococcus faecalis, Escherichia coli, Klebsiella pneumoniae, Staphylococcus aureus, S. epidermidis, Pseudomonas aeruginosa,* and *Candida albicans* (Novy, et al., 2015).

A 2007 study looked at the effects of eyebright eyedrops on newborns. Many premature babies have a reduced flow of tears in the first weeks after birth, leading to an increased risk of eye infection. Conventionally, these infections are treated with antibiotic eye drops containing neomycin. Recognising that this causes a risk to the newborn eye, as neomycin may be toxic to the baby's delicate eye tissues, the study investigated the use of eyebright eye drops containing sodium chloride in comparison to the conventional antibiotic eye drops. Sure enough, they found that the eyebright drops have such a strong antimicrobial action that the newborns treated with the herbal eye drops no longer required the risky antibiotic eye drops (Stoffel, et al., 2007).

Eyebright is effective in adult conjunctivitis, too. A study of eight patients with acute conjunctivitis showed that a single dose of eyebright eye drops relieved symptoms of itchiness, redness, weeping secretions, scratchiness, and puffy eyelids. Almost all of the participants experienced complete resolution of the condition within one week! Tolerability to the eye drops was very good – only three patients experienced mild reactions after seven days of continually using the eye drops, and one after 14 days. The researchers noted that this corresponded to the normal course of illness and was probably not a side effect of the eyebright, given that there were no undesirable adverse events from the eye drops occurring during the entire trial (Stoss, et al., 2000).

Goldenseal

Goldenseal eye baths have been traditionally used to treat conjunctivitis and **blepharitis**, but there is no experimental data available to back up this traditional use. We do know that goldenseal is rich in berberine, a strong antibacterial agent. However, it may be *too* strong.

CAUTION: A 2007 trial showed that the berberine derived from goldenseal is phototoxic to cells of the human lens – this means that caution must be used when applying goldenseal topically with eye baths or eye drops. Do not expose the eyes to bright sunlight after using goldenseal, as this may cause permanent damage to the lens of the eye (Chignell, et al., 2007).

Turmeric

Curcumin, an active and powerful constituent of turmeric, has anti-allergic, antimicrobial, and anti-inflammatory properties. Extracts of curcumin and whole turmeric may reduce the frequency and severity of seasonal allergic conjunctivitis and its antimicrobial properties may also treat infective cases. Taking turmeric orally can strengthen the immune system from the inside out, but topical application may work well, too. There aren't many studies on the effects of topical turmeric in conjunctivitis, but a proprietary herbal eye drop blend that included 1.3% turmeric was shown to relieve the symptoms of acute conjunctivitis (Biswas, et al., 2001).

A FINAL WORD…

I hope you have found this book informative and useful. If you do decide to take a nutritional supplement for your eyes, take a look at the **Vision Defender** range from Intelligent Formula.

Vision Defender supplements are:

- Proudly Made in the UK

- Premium Quality to Strict GMP (Good Manufacturing Practice) in MHRA (Medicines and Healthcare products Regulatory Agency) inspected premises

- Backed by Science

- Trusted by Thousands

Simply head over to VisionDefender.co.uk to find out more. If you can't find what you're looking for there, simply make contact via the website and let us know what you're after. We'd love to hear from you!

To get free updates of this book and special reader offers for Vision Defender eye-care supplements, go to www.VisionDefender.co.uk/eye-book

APPENDIX 1:
AMSLER GRID

Do you suffer from macular degeneration?

Use this handy Amsler Grid to help monitor and detect changes to your vision.

Procedure:

1. If you usually wear reading glasses, make sure you are wearing them.

2. Hold the grid at normal reading distance, about 30cm (12 inches) from your eyes.

3. Cover one eye and look at the central dot. Make sure you can see the entire grid.

4. If any lines look distorted, blurry, wavy, or have gaps, write down what you see.

5. Repeat with your other eye.

6. If any of these changes are new, **contact your optician or eye doctor immediately.**

Note: The Amsler Grid does not replace regular comprehensive eye-tests by your eyecare practitioner.

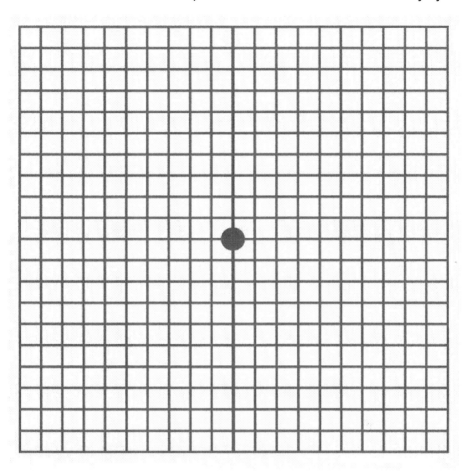

REFERENCES

Age-Related Eye Disease Study Research Group (2001) A randomised, placebo-controlled, clinical trial of high-dose supplementation with vitamins C and E, beta carotene, and zinc for age-related macular degeneration and vision loss: AREDS report no. 8. *Arch Ophthalmol., 119:10,* 1417 – 1436. https://www.ncbi.nlm.nih.gov/pubmed/11594942/

Age-Related Eye Disease Study 2 (AREDS2) Research Group (2013) Lutein + Zeaxanthin and Omega-3 Fatty Acids for Age-Related Macular Degeneration: The Age-Related Eye Disease Study 2 (AREDS2) Randomized Clinical Trial. *JAMA. 309(19),* 2005–2015. https://jamanetwork.com/journals/jama/fullarticle/1684847

Age-Related Eye Disease Study 2 (AREDS2) Research Group, et al. (2013) Lutein/zeaxanthin for the treatment of age-related cataract: AREDS2 randomized trial report no. 4. *J Ophthalmol., 131:7,* 843 – 850. https://www.ncbi.nlm.nih.gov/pubmed/23645227/

Albert, B., et al. (2013) Oxidation of Marine Omega-3 Supplements and Human Health. *BioMed Research International,* vol. 2013, Article ID 464921, 8 pages. https://www.hindawi.com/journals/bmri/2013/464921/

Alves, M., et al. (2005) Increased expression of advanced glycation end-products and their receptor, and activation of nuclear factor kappa-B in lacrimal glands of diabetic rats. *Diabetologia, 48:12,* 2675 – 2681. https://www.ncbi.nlm.nih.gov/pubmed/16283249

Aoki, A., et al. (2016) Dietary n-3 Fatty Acid, α-Tocopherol, Zinc, vitamin D, vitamin C, and β-carotene are Associated with Age-

Related Macular Degeneration in Japan. *Sci Rep., 6,* 20723. https://www.ncbi.nlm.nih.gov/pmc/articles/PMC4742947/

Ariano, R. (2015) Efficacy of a novel food supplement in the relief of the signs and symptoms of seasonal allergic rhinitis and in the reduction of the consumption of anti-allergic drugs. *Acta Biomed., 86:1,* 53 – 58. https://www.ncbi.nlm.nih.gov/pubmed/25948028

Aronow, M. E. & Chew, E. Y. (2014) AREDS2: Perspectives, Recommendations, and Unanswered Questions. *Curr Opin Ophthalmol., 25:3,* 186 – 190. https://www.ncbi.nlm.nih.gov/pmc/articles/PMC4096000/

Bae, S. H., et al. (2016) Vitamin D Supplementation for Patients with Dry Eye Syndrome Refractory to Conventional Treatment. *Sci Rep., 6,* 33083. https://www.ncbi.nlm.nih.gov/pmc/articles/PMC5048427/

Bernstein, P. F., et al. (2001) Identification and quantitation of carotenoids and their metabolites in the tissues of the human eye. *Exp Eye Res.,* 72(3), 215 – 23. https://www.ncbi.nlm.nih.gov/pubmed/11180970

Bhargava, R., et al. (2013) A randomized controlled trial of omega-3 fatty acids in dry eye syndrome. *Int J Ophthalmol., 6,* 811-816. https://www.ncbi.nlm.nih.gov/pubmed/24392330

Biswas, N. R., et al. (2001) Evaluation of Ophthacare eye drops--a herbal formulation in the management of various ophthalmic disorders. *Phytother Res., 15:7,* 618 – 620. https://www.ncbi.nlm.nih.gov/pubmed/11746845/

Boptom, S. L. M. & Braavedt, G. D. (2015) Impact of diabetes mellitus on the ocular surface: a review. *Clin Exp Ophthalmol., 44:4,* 278 – 288. https://onlinelibrary.wiley.com/doi/full/10.1111/ceo.12690

Bringmann, A., et al. (2016) Intake of dietary salt and drinking water: Implications for the development of age-related macular degeneration. *Mol Vis., 22,* 1437 – 1454. https://www.ncbi.nlm.nih.gov/pmc/articles/PMC5178186/

Calvo-Maroto, A. M., et al. (2014) Optical quality of the diabetic eye: a review. *Eye (Lond.), 28:11,* 1271 – 1280. https://www.ncbi.nlm.nih.gov/pmc/articles/PMC4274279/

Canter, P.H. & Ernst, E. (2004) Anthocyanosides of Vaccinium myrtillus (bilberry) for night vision-a systematic review of placebo-controlled trials. *Surv Ophthalmol., 49*, 38–50. https://www.ncbi.nlm.nih.gov/pubmed/14711439

Cardinault, N., et al. (2005) Lycopene but not lutein nor zeaxanthin decreases in serum and lipoproteins in age-related macular degeneration patients. *Clin Chim Acta, 357:1*, 34 – 42. https://www.ncbi.nlm.nih.gov/pubmed/15963792

Chambial, S., et al. (2013) Vitamin C in Disease Prevention and Cure: An Overview. *Indian J Clin Biochem., 28:4*, 314 – 328. https://www.ncbi.nlm.nih.gov/pmc/articles/PMC3783921/

Chandorkar, A. G., et al. (1980) Electrolyte composition in normal and cataractous lenses. *Indian Journal of Ophthalmology, 28:3*, 135 – 138. http://www.ijo.in/article.asp?issn=0301-4738;year=1980;volume=28;issue=3;spage=135;epage=138;aulast=Chandorkar

Chasan-Taber, L., et al. (1999) A prospective study of carotenoid and vitamin A intakes and risk of cataract extraction in US women. *Am J Clin Nutr., 70:4*, 509 – 516. https://www.ncbi.nlm.nih.gov/pubmed/10500020/

Chen, M., et al. (2010) Curcumin protects against hyperosmoticity-induced IL-1beta elevation in human corneal epithelial cell via MAPK pathways. *Exp Eye Res.* 90:3, 437 – 443. https://www.ncbi.nlm.nih.gov/pubmed/20026325/

Chen, X., et al. (2014) Diabetes Mellitus and Risk of Age-Related Macular Degeneration: A Systematic Review and Meta-Analysis. *PLoS ONE., 9:9.* https://www.ncbi.nlm.nih.gov/pmc/articles/PMC4169602/

Chignell, C. F., et al. (2007) Photochemistry and photocytotoxicity of alkaloids from Goldenseal (Hydrastis canadensis L.) 3: effect on human lens and retinal pigment epithelial cells. *Photochem Photobiol., 83:4*, 938 – 943. https://www.ncbi.nlm.nih.gov/pubmed/17645667

Chiu, C. J., et al. (2006) Dietary glycemic index and carbohydrate in relation to early age-related macular degeneration. *Am J Clin Nutr., 83:4*, 880 – 886. https://www.ncbi.nlm.nih.gov/

pubmed/16600942

Chiu, C. J., et al. (2007) Dietary carbohydrate and the progression of age-related macular degeneration: a prospective study from the Age-Related Eye Disease Study. *Am J Clin Nutr., 86:4,* 1210 – 1218. https://www.ncbi.nlm.nih.gov/pubmed/17921404

Chiu, C. J., et al. (2010) Dietary Carbohydrate in Relation to Cortical and Nuclear Lens Opacities in the Melbourne Visual Impairment Project. *Invest Ophthalmol Vis Sci., 51:6,* 2897 – 2905. https://www.ncbi.nlm.nih.gov/pmc/articles/PMC2891456/

Chiu, C. J. & Taylor, A. (2007) Nutritional antioxidants and age-related cataract and maculopathy. *Exp Eye Res., 84:2,* 229 – 245. https://www.ncbi.nlm.nih.gov/pubmed/16879819/

Chung, S. H., et al. (2012) Curcumin suppresses ovalbumin-induced allergic conjunctivitis. *Mol Vis., 18,* 1966- 1972. https://www.ncbi.nlm.nih.gov/pubmed/22876123/

Christen, W. G., et al. (2009) Folic Acid, Vitamin B6, and Vitamin B12 in Combination and Age-related Macular Degeneration in a Randomized Trial of Women. *Arch Intern Med., 169:4,* 335 – 341. https://www.ncbi.nlm.nih.gov/pmc/articles/PMC2648137/

Christen, W. G., et al. (2010) Age-related Cataract in a Randomized Trial of Vitamins E and C in Men. *Arch Ophthalmol., 128:11,* 1397 – 1405. https://www.ncbi.nlm.nih.gov/pmc/articles/PMC3051399/

Christen, W. G., et al. (2010) Vitamin E and Age-related Macular Degeneration in a Randomized Trial of Women. *Ophthalmology., 117:6,* 1163 – 1168. https://www.ncbi.nlm.nih.gov/pmc/articles/PMC2881167/

Chu, W., et al. (2011) *Bilberry.* Herbal Medicine: Biomolecular and Clinical Aspects. 2nd edition. https://www.ncbi.nlm.nih.gov/books/NBK92770/

Churchward, C. P., et al. (2017) Prevention of Ophthalmia Neonatorum Caused by *Neisseria gonorrhoeae* Using a Fatty Acid-Based Formulation. MB*io., 8:4,* https://www.ncbi.nlm.nih.gov/pmc/articles/PMC5527305/

Cumming, R. G., et al. (2000) Dietary sodium intake and cataract:

the Blue Mountains Eye Study. *Am J Epidemiol., 151:6,* 642 – 646. https://www.ncbi.nlm.nih.gov/pubmed/10733045

Dadaci, Z., et al. (2014) Plasma vitamin D and serum total immunoglobulin E levels in patients with seasonal allergic conjunctivitis. *Acta Ophthalmol., 92:6,* e443 – 446. https://www.ncbi.nlm.nih.gov/pubmed/24667068

Demmig-Adams, B. & Adams R. B. (2013) Eye Nutrition in Context: Mechanisms, Implementation, and Future Directions. *Nutrients., 5:7,* 2483 – 2501. https://www.ncbi.nlm.nih.gov/pmc/articles/PMC3738983/

Deng, H. W., et al. (2016) Effect of Bilberry Extract on Development of Form-Deprivation Myopia in the Guinea Pig. *J Ocul Pharmacol Ther., 32:4,* 196 – 202. https://www.ncbi.nlm.nih.gov/pubmed/26982283

de Souza, C. O., et al. (2018) Is Palmitoleic Acid a Plausible Nonpharmacological Strategy to Prevent or Control Chronic Metabolic and Inflammatory Disorders? *Mol Nutr Food Res., 62:1.* https://www.ncbi.nlm.nih.gov/pubmed/28980402

Duignan, E., et al. (2015) Ophthalmic Manifestations of Vitamin A and D Deficiency in Two Autistic Teenagers: Case Reports and a Review of the Literature. *Case Rep Ophthalmol., 6:1,* 24 – 29. https://www.ncbi.nlm.nih.gov/pmc/articles/PMC4327555/

Etheridge, A. S., et al. (2007) An in vitro evaluation of cytochrome P450 inhibition and P-glycoprotein interaction with goldenseal, Ginkgo biloba, grape seed, milk thistle, and ginseng extracts and their constituents. *Planta Med., 73:8,* 731 – 741. https://www.ncbi.nlm.nih.gov/pubmed/17611934

Etminan, M., et al. (2008) Use of statins and angiotensin converting enzyme inhibitors (ACE-Is) and the risk of age-related macular degeneration: nested case-control study. *Curr Drug Saf., 3:1,* 24 – 26. https://www.ncbi.nlm.nih.gov/pubmed/18690977

Fischer, P. W., et al. (1981) The effect of dietary zinc on intestinal copper absorption. *Am J Clin Nutr., 34:9,* 1670 – 1675. https://www.ncbi.nlm.nih.gov/pubmed/7282591

Francisco, B., et al. (2015) Oxidative Stress in Myopia. *Oxid Med*

Cell Longev., 2015. https://www.ncbi.nlm.nih.gov/pmc/articles/PMC4397465/

Gasper, A. Z., et al. (1995) The influence of magnesium on visual field and peripheral vasospasm in glaucoma. *Ophthalmologica., 209:1,* 11 – 13. https://www.ncbi.nlm.nih.gov/pubmed/7715920/

Gillery, P. (2001) Advanced glycation end products (AGEs), free radicals and diabetes. *J Soc Biol., 195:4,* 387 – 390. https://www.ncbi.nlm.nih.gov/pubmed/11938555

García-Closas, R., et al. (2004) Dietary sources of vitamin C, vitamin E and specific carotenoids in Spain. *Br J Nutr., 91:6,* 1005 – 1011. https://www.ncbi.nlm.nih.gov/pubmed/15182404

Gratton, S. M. & Lam, B. L. (2014) Visual loss and optic nerve head swelling in thiamine deficiency without prolonged dietary deficiency. *Clin Ophthalmol., 8,* 1021 – 1024. https://www.ncbi.nlm.nih.gov/pmc/articles/PMC4039400

Gupta, S. K., et al. (2003) Lycopene attenuates oxidative stress induced experimental cataract development: an in vitro and in vivo study. *Nutrition., 19:9,* 794 – 799. https://www.ncbi.nlm.nih.gov/pubmed/12921892

Gurley, B. J., et al. (2008a) Supplementation with goldenseal (Hydrastis canadensis), but not kava kava (Piper methysticum), inhibits human CYP3A activity in vivo. *Clin Pharmacol Ther., 83:1,* 61 – 69. https://www.ncbi.nlm.nih.gov/pubmed/17495878

Gurley, B. J., et al. (2008b) Clinical assessment of CYP2D6-mediated herb-drug interactions in humans: effects of milk thistle, black cohosh, goldenseal, kava kava, St. John's wort, and Echinacea. *Mol Nutr Food Res., 52:7,* 755 – 763. https://www.ncbi.nlm.nih.gov/pubmed/18214849

Hashimoto, H., et al. (2013) Effects of astaxanthin on antioxidation in human aqueous humour. *J Clin Biochem Nutr., 53 – 1,* 1 – 7. https://www.ncbi.nlm.nih.gov/pmc/articles/PMC3705160/

Ho, L., et al. (2011) Reducing the genetic risk of age-related macular degeneration with dietary antioxidants, zinc, and ω-3 fatty acids: the Rotterdam study. Arch Ophthalmol., 129:6, 758 – 766.

https://www.ncbi.nlm.nih.gov/pubmed/21670343/

Hoffman, H., et al. (1988) Zinc-induced copper deficiency. *Gastroenterology, 94:2,* 508 – 512. https://www.ncbi.nlm.nih.gov/pubmed/3335323

Hom, M. & De Land, P. (2006) Self-reported dry eyes and diabetic history. *Optometry., 77:11,* 554 – 558. https://www.ncbi.nlm.nih.gov/pubmed/17145567/

Howes, K. A., et al. (2004) Receptor for advanced glycation end products and age-related macular degeneration. *Invest Ophthalmol Vis Sci., 45:10,* 3713 – 3720. https://www.ncbi.nlm.nih.gov/pubmed/15452081

Hu, B., et al. (2011) Application of Lutein and Zeaxanthin in non-proliferative diabetic retinopathy. *Int J Ophthalmol., 4:3,* 303 – 306. https://www.ncbi.nlm.nih.gov/pmc/articles/PMC3340817/

Hu, Y. H., et al. (2012) Curcumin inhibits proliferation of human lens epithelial cells: a proteomic analysis. *J Zhejiang Univ Sci B., 13:5,* 402 – 407. https://www.ncbi.nlm.nih.gov/pubmed/22556179/

Huibi, X., et al. (2001) Prevention of axial elongation in myopia by the trace element zinc. *Biol Trace Elem Res., 79:1,* 39 – 47. https://www.ncbi.nlm.nih.gov/pubmed/11318236

Januleviciene, I., et al. (2012) Ophthalmic Drug Delivery in Glaucoma—A Review. *Pharmaceutics., 4:1,* 243 – 251. https://www.ncbi.nlm.nih.gov/pmc/articles/PMC3834898/

Jayawardena, R., et al. (2012) Effects of zinc supplementation on diabetes mellitus: a systematic review and meta-analysis. *Diabetic and Metabolic Syndrome., 4:13.* https://dmsjournal.biomedcentral.com/articles/10.1186/1758-5996-4-13

Johnson, L. E. (2016) Vitamin D. *Merck Manual Database,* http://www.merckmanuals.com/en-pr/professional/nutritional-disorders/vitamin-deficiency,-dependency,-and-toxicity/vitamin-d

Kajita, M., et al. (2009) The Effects of a Dietary Supplement Containing Astaxanthin on the Accommodation Function of the Eye in Middle-aged and Older People. *Medical Consultation*

& *New Remedies., 46:3.* http://www.flex-news-food.com/files/bioreal031209.pdf

Kamiya, K., et al. (2013) Effect of fermented bilberry extracts on visual outcomes in eyes with myopia: a prospective, randomized, placebo-controlled study. *J Ocul Pharmacol Ther., 29:3*, 356 – 359. https://www.ncbi.nlm.nih.gov/pubmed/23113643

Kang, K. D., et al. (2010) Sulbutiamine counteracts trophic factor deprivation induced apoptotic cell death in transformed retinal ganglion cells. *Neurochem Res., 35:11*, 1828 – 1839. https://www.ncbi.nlm.nih.gov/pubmed/20809085/

Khazaeni, L. M. (2017) Cataract. *Merck Manual Online Professional.* https://www.msdmanuals.com/en-au/professional/eye-disorders/cataract/cataract

Kim, H. T., et al. (2016) The Relationship between Vitamin D and Glaucoma: A Kangbuk Samsung Health Study. *Korean J Ophthalmol., 30:6*, 426 – 433. https://www.ncbi.nlm.nih.gov/pmc/articles/PMC5156616/

Klein, R., et al. (2014) Vasodilators, blood pressure-lowering medications, and age-related macular degeneration: the Beaver Dam Eye Study. *Ophthalmology, 121:8*, 1604 – 1611. https://www.ncbi.nlm.nih.gov/pubmed/24793737/

Kono, K., et al. (2014) Effect of Multiple Dietary Supplement Containing Lutein,
Astaxanthin, Cyanidin-3-Glucoside, and DHA on Accommodative Ability. *Curr Med Chem., 14:2*, 114 – 125. https://www.ncbi.nlm.nih.gov/pmc/articles/PMC4997915/

Koo, H., et al. (2012) Ocular Surface Discomfort and Demodex: Effect of Tea Tree Oil Eyelid Scrub in Demodex Blepharitis. *J Korean Med Sci., 27:12*, 1574 – 1578. https://www.ncbi.nlm.nih.gov/pmc/articles/PMC3524441/

Koushan, K., et al. (2013) The Role of Lutein in Eye-Related Disease. *Nutrients., 5:5*, 1823 – 1839. https://www.ncbi.nlm.nih.gov/pmc/articles/PMC3708350/

Kruk, J., et al. (2015) The Role Oxidative Stress in the Pathogenesis of Eye Diseases: Current Status and a Dual Role of Physical Activity. *Mini Rev Med Chem., 16:3*, 241 – 257. https://

www.ncbi.nlm.nih.gov/pubmed/26586128

Kumar, P. A., et al. (2005) Modulation of alpha-crystallin chaperone activity in diabetic rat lens by curcumin. *Mol Vis., 11*, 561 – 568. https://www.ncbi.nlm.nih.gov/pubmed/16088325

Langman, M. J. S., et al. (2005) Systemic hypertension and glaucoma: mechanisms in common and co-occurrence. *Br J Ophthalmol., 89:8*, 960 – 963. https://www.ncbi.nlm.nih.gov/pmc/articles/PMC1772770/

Layana, A. G., et al. (2017) Vitamin D and Age-Related Macular Degeneration. *Nutrients., 9:10*, 1120. https://www.ncbi.nlm.nih.gov/pmc/articles/PMC5691736/

Li, B., et al. (2010) Studies on the singlet oxygen scavenging mechanism of human macular pigment. Arch Biochem Biophys., 504:1, 56 – 60. https://www.ncbi.nlm.nih.gov/pubmed/20678467

Li, M., et al. (2011) The effect of caffeine on intraocular pressure: a systematic review and meta-analysis. *Graefe's Archive for Clinical and Experimental Ophthalmology., 249:3*, 435 – 442. https://link.springer.com/article/10.1007%2Fs00417-010-1455-1

Lim, E. L., et al. (2011) Reversal of type 2 diabetes: normalisation of beta cell function in association with decreased pancreas and liver triacylglycerol. *Diabetologia, 54:10*, 2506 – 2514. https://www.ncbi.nlm.nih.gov/pmc/articles/PMC3168743/

Liu, J., et al. (2010) Pathogenic role of *Demodex* mites in blepharitis. *Curr Opin Allergy Clin Immunol., 10:5*, 505 – 510. https://www.ncbi.nlm.nih.gov/pmc/articles/PMC2946818/

Lobo, V., et al. (2010) Free radicals, antioxidants and functional foods: Impact on human health. *Pharmacogn Review., 4:8*, 118 – 126. https://www.ncbi.nlm.nih.gov/pmc/articles/PMC3249911/

Loughman, J., et al. (2012) The impact of macular pigment augmentation on visual performance using different carotenoid formulations. *Invest Ophthalmol Vis Sci., 53:12*, 7871 – 7880. https://www.ncbi.nlm.nih.gov/pubmed/23132800/

Ma, L., et al. (2016) Lutein, Zeaxanthin and Meso-zeaxanthin Supplementation Associated with Macular Pigment Optical Density. *Nutrients.*, *8:7*, 426. https://www.ncbi.nlm.nih.gov/pmc/articles/PMC4963902/

Macsai, M. S. (2008) The Role of Omega-3 Dietary Supplementation in Blepharitis and Meibomian Gland Dysfunction (An AOS Thesis). *Trans Am Ophthalmol Soc.*, *106*, 336 – 356. https://www.ncbi.nlm.nih.gov/pmc/articles/PMC2646454/

Maher, T. N. (2018) The use of tea tree oil in treating blepharitis and meibomian gland dysfunction. *Oman J Ophthalmol.*, *11:1*, 11 – 15. https://www.ncbi.nlm.nih.gov/pmc/articles/PMC5848340/

Manikandan, R., et al. (2010) Curcumin prevents free radical-mediated cataractogenesis through modulations in lens calcium. *Free Radic Biol Med.*, *48:4*, 483 – 492. https://www.ncbi.nlm.nih.gov/pubmed/19932168/

Mares, J. (2017) Lutein and Zeaxanthin Isomers in Eye Health and Disease. *Annu Rev Nutr.*, *36*, 571 – 602. https://www.ncbi.nlm.nih.gov/pmc/articles/PMC5611842/

McCarty, C. A., et al. (2001) Risk factors for age-related maculopathy: the Visual Impairment Project. *Arch Ophthalmol.*, *119:10*, 1455 – 1462. https://www.ncbi.nlm.nih.gov/pubmed/11594944/

McNeil J.J., et al. (2004) Vitamin E supplementation and cataract: randomized controlled trial. *Ophthalmology.*, *111:1*, 75-84. https://www.ncbi.nlm.nih.gov/pubmed/14711717

Michael, R. & Bron, A. J. (2011) The ageing lens and cataract: a model of normal and pathological ageing. *Philos Trans R Soc Lond B Biol Sci.*, *366*, 1278 – 1292. https://www.ncbi.nlm.nih.gov/pmc/articles/PMC3061107/

Mirsamadi, M., et al. (2004) Comparative study of serum Na+ and K+ levels in senile cataract patients and normal individuals. *Int J Med Sci.*, *1:3*, 165 – 169. https://www.ncbi.nlm.nih.gov/pmc/articles/PMC1074711/#B5

Moïse, M. M., et al. (2012) Role of Mediterranean diet, tropical vegetables rich in antioxidants, and sunlight exposure in blindness, cataract and glaucoma among African type 2 diabetics. *Int J Ophthalmol.*, *5:2*, 231 – 237. https://www.ncbi.nlm.nih.gov/pubmed/22762057

Mordente, A., et al. (2011) Lycopene and cardiovascular diseases: an update. *Curr Med Chem., 18:8,* 1446 – 1463. https://www.ncbi.nlm.nih.gov/pubmed/21291369

Murugan, P. & Pari, L. (2006) Antioxidant effect of tetrahydrocurcumin in streptozotocin-nicotinamide induced diabetic rats. *Life Sci., 79:18,* 1720 – 1728. https://www.ncbi.nlm.nih.gov/pubmed/16806281/

Müskens, R. P., et al. (2007) Systemic antihypertensive medication and incident open-angle glaucoma. *Ophthalmology., 114:12,* 2221 – 2226. https://www.ncbi.nlm.nih.gov/pubmed/17568677/

Mutti, D. O., et al. (2002) Parental myopia, near work, school achievement, and children's refractive error. *Invest Ophthalmol Vis Sci., 43:12,* 3633 – 3640. https://www.ncbi.nlm.nih.gov/pubmed/12454029/

Mutti, D. O. & Marks, A. R. (2011) Blood Levels of Vitamin D in Teens and Young Adults with Myopia. *Optom Vis Sci., 88:3,* 377 – 382. https://www.ncbi.nlm.nih.gov/pmc/articles/PMC3044787/

Nakamura, S., et al. (2017) Restoration of Tear Secretion in a Murine Dry Eye Model by Oral Administration of Palmitoleic Acid. *Nutrients., 9:4,* 364. https://www.ncbi.nlm.nih.gov/pmc/articles/PMC5409703/

Nagaki, Y., et al. (2002) Effects of astaxanthin on accommodation, critical flicker fusion, and pattern visual evoked potential in visual display terminal workers. *OAI.* https://www.researchgate.net/publication/47294524_Effects_of_astaxanthin_on_accommodation_critical_flicker_fusion_and_pattern_visual_evoked_potential_in_visual_display_terminal_workers

NHS (2017) Sodium chloride (salt). https://www.nhs.uk/conditions/vitamins-and-minerals/others/#sodium-chloride-salt Last accessed: 25th July 2018

Nolan, J. M., et al. (2013) What is meso-zeaxanthin, and where does it come from? *Eye (Lond.)., 27:8,* 899 – 905. https://www.ncbi.nlm.nih.gov/pmc/articles/PMC3740325/

Novy, P., et al. (2015) Composition and Antimicrobial Activity of Euphrasia rostkoviana Hayne Essential Oil. *Evid Based Complement Altern Med.*, 734101. https://www.ncbi.nlm.nih.gov/pubmed/26000025

Oleñik, A., et al. (2014) Benefits of omega-3 fatty acid dietary supplementation on health-related quality of life in patients with meibomian gland dysfunction. *Clin Ophthalmol.*, 8, 831 – 836. https://www.ncbi.nlm.nih.gov/pmc/articles/PMC4010636/#b22-opth-8-831

Olmedilla, B., et al. (2003) Lutein, but not alpha-tocopherol, supplementation improves visual function in patients with age-related cataracts: a 2-y double-blind, placebo-controlled pilot study. *Nutrition.*, 19:1, 21 – 24. https://www.ncbi.nlm.nih.gov/pubmed/12507634/

Otsuka, T., et al. (2013) The Protective Effects of a Dietary Carotenoid, Astaxanthin, Against Light-Induced Retinal Damage. *J Pharmacol Sci.*, 123, 209 – 218. https://www.jstage.jst.go.jp/article/jphs/123/3/123_13066FP/_pdf/-char/en

Paduch, R., et al. (2014) Assessment of Eyebright (Euphrasia Officinalis L.) Extract Activity in Relation to Human Corneal Cells Using *In Vitro* Tests. *Balkan Med J.*, 31:1, 29 – 36. https://www.ncbi.nlm.nih.gov/pmc/articles/PMC4115993/

Parisi, V., et al. (2014) Effects of Coenzyme Q10 in Conjunction With Vitamin E on Retinal-evoked and Cortical-evoked Responses in Patients With Open-angle Glaucoma. *Journal of Glaucoma,* 23:6, 391 – 404. https://insights.ovid.com/crossref?an=00061198-201408000-00011

Parodi, M. B., et al. (2016) Nutritional Supplementation in Age Related Macular-Degeneration. *Retina.,* 36, 111 9 – 1125. https://journals.lww.com/retinajournal/Abstract/2016/06000/NUTRITIONAL_SUPPLEMENTATION_IN_AGE_RELATED_MACULAR.11.aspx

Peppa, M., et al. (2003) Glucose, Advanced Glycation End Products, and Diabetes Complications: What Is New and What Works. *Clinical Diabetes,* 21:4, 186 – 187. http://clinical.diabetesjournals.org/content/21/4/186.full

Petyaev, I. M. (2016) Lycopene Deficiency in Ageing and Cardiovascular Disease. *Oxid Med Cell Longev., 2016.* https://www.ncbi.nlm.nih.gov/pmc/articles/PMC4736775/

Pham-Huy, L. A., et al. (2008) Free Radicals, Antioxidants in Disease and Health. *Int J Biomed Sci., 4:2,* 89 – 96. https://www.ncbi.nlm.nih.gov/pmc/articles/PMC3614697/

Pollack, A., et al. (1985) Inhibitory effect of lycopene on cataract development in galactosemic rats. *Metab Pediatr Syst Ophthalmol., 19:20,* 31 – 36. https://www.ncbi.nlm.nih.gov/pubmed/11548783

Privett, B. & Mahajan, V. B. (2011) Vitamin A Deficiency and Nyctalopia: 55-year-old male with gradual onset of night blindness. *EyeRounds.org.* https://webeye.ophth.uiowa.edu/eyeforum/cases/130-vitamin-a-deficiency.htm

Ramdas, W. D., et al. (2012) Nutrient intake and risk of open-angle glaucoma: the Rotterdam Study. *Eur J Epidemiol., 27:5,* 385 – 393. https://www.ncbi.nlm.nih.gov/pmc/articles/PMC3374099/

Ramdas, W. D., et al. (2018) The Effect of Vitamins on Glaucoma: A Systematic Review and Meta-Analysis. *Nutrients., 10:3,* 359. http://www.mdpi.com/2072-6643/10/3/359/htm

Rasmussen, H. M., et al. (2013) Nutrients for the aging eye. *Clin Interv Aging., 8,* 741 – 748. https://www.ncbi.nlm.nih.gov/pmc/articles/PMC3693724/

Ravindran, R. D., et al. (2011) Inverse Association of Vitamin C with Cataract in Older People in India. *Ophthalmology., 118:10,* 1958 – 1965. https://www.ncbi.nlm.nih.gov/pmc/articles/PMC3185206

Reins, R. Y. & McDermott, A. M. (2015) Vitamin D: Implications for Ocular Disease and Therapeutic Potential. *Exp Eye Res., 134,* 101 – 110. https://www.ncbi.nlm.nih.gov/pmc/articles/PMC4426046

Richer, S. P. & Pizzimenti, J. J. (2013) The importance of vitamin D in systemic and ocular wellness. *J Optom., 6:3,* 124 – 133. https://www.ncbi.nlm.nih.gov/pmc/articles/PMC3880532/

Royal College of Ophthalmologists (2010) Cataract Surgery Guidelines. https://www.rcophth.ac.uk/wp-content/

uploads/2014/12/2010-SCI-069-Cataract-Surgery-Guidelines-2010-SEPTEMBER-2010-1.pdf Last accessed: 25th July 2018

SanGiovanni J. P., et al. (2007) The relationship of dietary lipid intake and age-related macular degeneration in a case-control study: AREDS Report No. 20. *Arch Ophthalmol. 125*, 671–679. https://www.ncbi.nlm.nih.gov/pubmed/17502507

SanGiovanni J. P., et al. (2009) ω-3 Long-Chain Polyunsaturated Fatty Acid Intake Inversely Associated With 12-Year Progression to Advanced Age-Related Macular Degeneration. *Arch Ophthalmol. 127(1)*, 109–116. https://jamanetwork.com/journals/jamaophthalmology/fullarticle/420997

Schleicher, M., et al. (2013) Diminishing Risk for Age-Related Macular Degeneration with Nutrition: A Current View. *Nutrients., 5:7*, 2405 – 2456. https://www.ncbi.nlm.nih.gov/pmc/articles/PMC3738980/

Sievert, M. (2017) Ions Electrolytes and Free Radicals. https://www.americorpshealth.biz/physiology/ions-electrolytes-and-free-radicals.html

Seddon, J. M., et al. (1994) Dietary carotenoids, vitamins A, C, and E, and advanced age-related macular degeneration. Eye Disease Case-Control Study Group. *JAMA., 272:18.* 1413 – 1420. https://www.ncbi.nlm.nih.gov/pubmed/7933422/

Seddon J. M., et al. (2006) Cigarette smoking, fish consumption, omega-3 fatty acid intake, and associations with age-related macular degeneration: the US Twin Study of Age-Related Macular Degeneration. *Arch Ophthalmol 124*, 995–1001. https://www.ncbi.nlm.nih.gov/pubmed/16832023

Sen, S. K., et al. (2008) Plasma Homocysteine, Folate and Vitamin B12 levels in senile cataract. *Indian J Clinic Biochem., 23:3*, 255 – 257. https://www.ncbi.nlm.nih.gov/pmc/articles/PMC3453456/

Sethu, S., et al. (2016) Correlation between tear fluid and serum vitamin D levels. *Eye Vis(Lond.), 3:1*, 22. https://www.ncbi.nlm.nih.gov/pmc/articles/PMC5009644/

Silverstone, B. Z. (1990) Effects of zinc and copper metabolism in highly myopic patients. *Ciba Found Symp., 155*, 210 – 217. https://

www.ncbi.nlm.nih.gov/pubmed/2088677

Simopoulus, A. P. (2002) The importance of the ratio of omega-6/omega-3 essential fatty acids. Biomed Pharmacother., 56:8, 365 – 379. https://www.ncbi.nlm.nih.gov/pubmed/12442909

Smailhodzic, D., et al. (2014) Zinc Supplementation Inhibits Complement Activation in Age-Related Macular Degeneration. *PLoS ONE.*, *9:11*, https://www.ncbi.nlm.nih.gov/pmc/articles/PMC4231060/

Sommerburg, O., et al. (1998) Fruits and vegetables that are sources for lutein and zeaxanthin: the macular pigment in human eyes. *Br J Ophthalmol.*, *82:8*, 907 – 910. https://www.ncbi.nlm.nih.gov/pmc/articles/PMC1722697/

Song, M., et al. (2015) Effects of lutein or lutein in combination with vitamin C on mRNA expression and activity of antioxidant enzymes and status of the antioxidant system in SD rats. *Lab Anim Res.*, *31:3*, 117 – 124. https://www.ncbi.nlm.nih.gov/pmc/articles/PMC4602078/

Souied E. H., et al. (2016) Omega-3 Fatty Acids and Age-Related Macular Degeneration. *Ophthalmic Res.*, *55*, 62-69. https://www.karger.com/Article/FullText/441359

Stoffel, L., et al. (2007) *Euphrasia* eye drops in newborns: a pilot project. *Switzerland Z Ganzheitsmed.*, *19:5*, 254 – 259. https://www.karger.com/Article/Abstract/283798

Stoss, M., et al. (2000) Prospective cohort trial of Euphrasia single-dose eye drops in conjunctivitis. *J Altern Complement Med.*, *6:6*, 499 – 508. https://www.ncbi.nlm.nih.gov/pubmed/11152054

Suryanarayana, P., et al. (2005) Curcumin and turmeric delay streptozotocin-induced diabetic cataract in rats. *Invest Ophthalmol Vis Sci.*, 46:6, 2092- 2099. https://iovs.arvojournals.org/article.aspx?articleid=2163736

Tan, J., et al. (2007) Carbohydrate nutrition, glycemic index, and the 10-y incidence of cataract. *The American Journal of Clinical Nutrition, 5:1*, 1502 – 1508. https://academic.oup.com/ajcn/article-abstract/86/5/1502/4650736?redirectedFrom=fulltext

Tan, J. S., et al. (2008) Dietary antioxidants and the long-term incidence of age-related macular degeneration: the Blue

Mountains Eye Study. *Ophthalmology., 115:2,* 334 – 341. https://www.ncbi.nlm.nih.gov/pubmed/17664009/

Tanaka, T., et al. (2012) Cancer chemoprevention by carotenoids. *Molecules., 17:3,* 3202 – 3242. https://www.ncbi.nlm.nih.gov/pubmed/22418926/

Taylor, H. R., et al. (2002) Vitamin E supplementation and macular degeneration: randomised controlled trial. *BMJ., 325:7354,* 11. https://www.ncbi.nlm.nih.gov/pmc/articles/PMC116664/

Tezel, G., et al. (2007) Accelerated aging in glaucoma: immunohistochemical assessment of advanced glycation end products in the human retina and optic nerve head. *Invest Ophthalmol Vis Sci., 48:3,* 1201 – 1211. https://www.ncbi.nlm.nih.gov/pubmed/17325164

The Dry Eye Assessment and Management Study Research Group (2018) n-3 Fatty Acid Supplementation for the Treatment of Dry Eye Disease. *The New England Journal of Medicine, 378,* 1681 – 1690. https://www.nejm.org/doi/full/10.1056/NEJMoa1709691

Tideman, J. W., et al. (2016) Low serum vitamin D is associated with axial length and risk of myopia in young children. *Eur J Epidemiol., 31:5,* 491 – 499. https://www.ncbi.nlm.nih.gov/pubmed/26955828

Valero, M. P., et al. (2002) Vitamin C is associated with reduced risk of cataract in a Mediterranean population. *J Nutr., 132:6,* 1299 – 1306. https://www.ncbi.nlm.nih.gov/pubmed/12042450

Vishwanathan, R., et al. (2013) A systematic review on zinc for the prevention and treatment of age-related macular degeneration. *Invest Ophthalmol Vis Sci., 54:6,* 3985 – 3998. https://www.ncbi.nlm.nih.gov/pubmed/23652490

Wang, S. Y., et al. (2013) Glaucoma and vitamins A, C, and E supplement intake and serum levels in a population-based sample of the United States. *Eye, 27:4,* 487 – 494. https://www.ncbi.nlm.nih.gov/pmc/articles/PMC3626010/

Wapnir, R. A. & Balkman, C. (1991) Inhibition of copper absorption by zinc. *Biological Trace Element Research., 29:3,* 193 – 202. https://link.springer.com/article/10.1007%2FBF03032677

Webb, B. F., et al. (2013) Prevalence of vitreous floaters in a community sample of smartphone users. *Int J Ophthalmol., 6:3*, 402 – 405. https://www.ncbi.nlm.nih.gov/pmc/articles/PMC3693028/

Weikel, K. A., et al. (2014) Nutritional modulation of cataract. *Nutr Rev, 72:1*, 30 – 47. https://www.ncbi.nlm.nih.gov/pmc/articles/PMC4097885/

Williams, K. A., et al. (2017) Association Between Myopia, Ultraviolet B Radiation Exposure, Serum Vitamin D Concentrations, and Genetic Polymorphisms in Vitamin D Metabolic Pathways in a Multicountry European Study. *JAMA Ophthalmology., 135:1*, 47 – 53. https://jamanetwork.com/journals/jamaophthalmology/fullarticle/2588252

Woodward, A. M., et al. (2014) Differential contribution of hypertonic electrolytes to corneal epithelial dysfunction. *Exp Eye Res., 100*, 98 – 100. https://www.ncbi.nlm.nih.gov/pmc/articles/PMC3889657/

Wu, J., et al. (2015) Intakes of Lutein, Zeaxanthin, and Other Carotenoids and Age-Related Macular Degeneration During 2 Decades of Prospective Follow-up. *JAMA Ophthalmol., 133:12*, 1415 – 1424. https://www.ncbi.nlm.nih.gov/pmc/articles/PMC5119484/

Yang, C. H., et al. (2017) Impact of oral vitamin D supplementation on the ocular surface in people with dry eye and/or low serum vitamin D. *Contact Lens and Anterior Eye.* http://dx.doi.org/10.1016/j.clae.2017.09.007

Yeh, P., et al. (2016) Astaxanthin Inhibits Expression of Retinal Oxidative Stress and Inflammatory Mediators in Streptozotocin-Induced Diabetic Rats. *PLoS One., 11:1*, https://www.ncbi.nlm.nih.gov/pmc/articles/PMC4713224/

Yu, X., et al. (2014) Hypertension and Risk of Cataract: A Meta-Analysis. *PLoS ONE., 9:12*, e114012. https://www.ncbi.nlm.nih.gov/pmc/articles/PMC4256215/

Yue, Y. K., et al. (2014) Neuroprotective effect of curcumin against oxidative damage in BV-2 microglia and high intraocular pressure animal model. J Ocul Pharmacol Ther. 3:8, 657-64. https://www.ncbi.nlm.nih.gov/pubmed/24963995/

Zafra-Stone, S., et al. (2007) Berry anthocyanins as novel antioxidants in human health and disease prevention. *Mol Nutr Food Res.*, *51*, 675–683.
https://www.ncbi.nlm.nih.gov/pubmed/17533652

Zarnowski, T., et al. (2012) A Ketogenic Diet May Offer Neuroprotection in Glaucoma and Mitochondrial Diseases of the Optic Nerve. *Med Hypothesis Discov Innov Ophthalmol.*, *1:3*, 45 – 49.
https://www.ncbi.nlm.nih.gov/pmc/articles/PMC3939735/

Zhang, Y., et al. (2015) Vitamin E and risk of age-related cataract: a meta-analysis. *Public Health Nutr.*, *18:15*, 2804 – 2814. https://www.ncbi.nlm.nih.gov/pubmed/25591715

Zhang, X., et al. (2016) Dry Eye Syndrome in Patients with Diabetes Mellitus: Prevalence, Etiology, and Clinical Characteristics. *J Ophthalmol.*, *26.* https://www.ncbi.nlm.nih.gov/pmc/articles/PMC4861815/

Zubaty, V., et al. (2008) Increased Advanced Glycation End-Products (AGEs) in Trabecular Meshwork of Patients With Primary and Secondary Glaucoma. *Investigative Ophthalmology & Visual Science.*, *49*, 1607. http://iovs.arvojournals.org/article.aspx?articleid=2377056

Printed in Great Britain
by Amazon